Combating Nutritional Blindness in Children

(Pergamon Policy Studies—57)

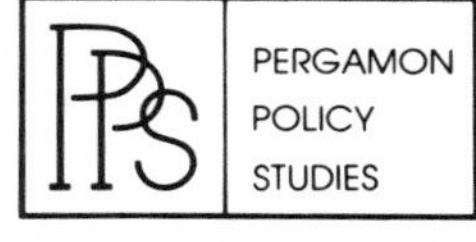

ON SOCIO-ECONOMIC DEVELOPMENT

Combating Nutritional Blindness in Children

A Case Study of Technical Assistance in Indonesia

Carl Fritz

Pergamon Press
NEW YORK • OXFORD • TORONTO • SYDNEY • FRANKFURT • PARIS

Pergamon Press Offices:

U.S.A.	Pergamon Press Inc., Maxwell House, Fairview Park, Elmsford, New York 10523, U.S.A.
U.K.	Pergamon Press Ltd., Headington Hill Hall, Oxford OX3 0BW, England
CANADA	Pergamon of Canada Ltd., 150 Consumers Road, Willowdale, Ontario M2J 1P9, Canada
AUSTRALIA	Pergamon Press (Aust) Pty. Ltd., P O Box 544, Potts Point, NSW 2011, Australia
FRANCE	Pergamon Press SARL, 24 rue des Ecoles, 75240 Paris, Cedex 05, France
FEDERAL REPUBLIC OF GERMANY	Pergamon Press GmbH, 6242 Kronberg/Taunus, Pferdstrasse 1, Federal Republic of Germany

Library of Congress Cataloging in Publication Data

Fritz, Carl, 1923-
Combatting nutritional blindness in children.

(Pergamon policy studies)
Bibliography: p.
Includes index.
1. Children, Blind—Services for—Indonesia.
2. Blindness—Indonesia—Nutritional aspects.
3. Blindness—Indonesia—Prevention—International cooperation. 4. Nutrition disorders in children—Indonesia. 5. Medical assistance, American—Indonesia.
6. Technical assistance, American—Indonesia.
I. Title.
RE48.2.C5F74 1979 617.7'12'071 79-15185
ISBN 0-08-024636-2

Printed in the United States of America

... The project might well serve as an example of what can be accomplished in a short time when gifted leadership, co-operation, dedication and adequate resources can be suitably harmonized together.

An Evaluation Report
June 4, 1978

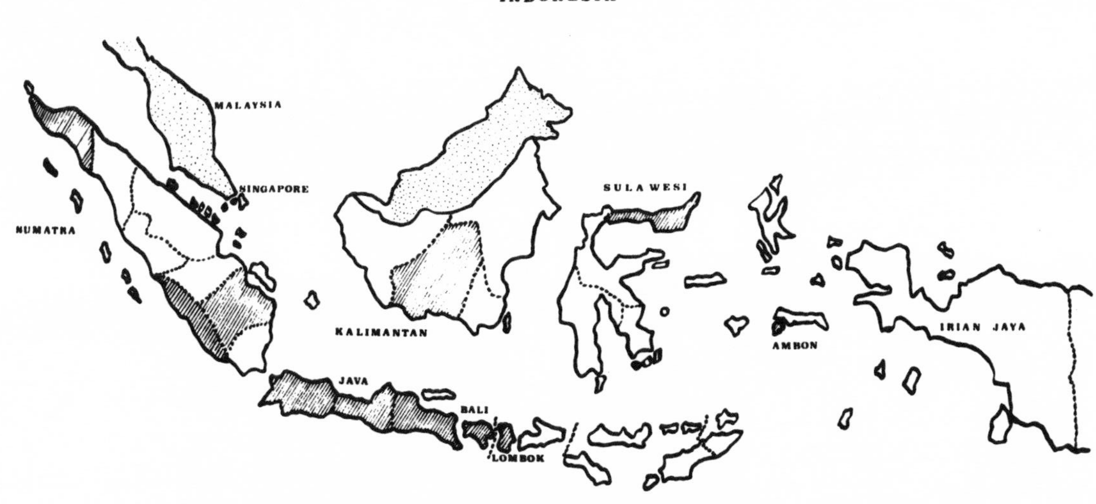

Results of Study IV showing critical areas of nutritional eye disease in children (Sumatera:Sumatra; Jawa:Java; Kalimantan:Borneo; Sulawesi:Celebes; N. T. T.:East Nusa Tenggara; Maluku:Maluccas).

Contents

Preface

> If a man has lived with a problem, reflected upon it, studied it, has been trained to deal with the problem, then he is morally committed to expressing an opinion. (1)

As a long-term student and participant in the processes of international technical assistance (TA), I have been distressed by the lack of understanding which exists among many administrators of foreign aid and their political overseers. Assignment by the Helen Keller International organization to the Indonesian Nutritional Blindness Research Project has given me an opportunity to document fully the problems and triumphs of a TA project and to satisfy myself that principles which I espouse are applicable. Helen Keller International, while jointly responsible with the Indonesian Government for the conduct of the project under review, has played no part in the preparation of this case study of technical assistance. I performed the writing on my own time as a work of love. Any opinions, findings, conclusions, or recommendations expressed herein are those of the author, arrived at independently of my current employer, Helen Keller International (HKI), and the United States Agency for International Development, whose contract with HKI made possible the project described in the case study.

I recognize that some of my case study comments may be considered as criticism of the Agency for International Development (AID) and the Indonesian government. To catalog problems is not meant to condemn, but instead to underline the need for new and more effective policies and procedures. I have tried to record my experiences and observations as I saw them. Every organization and government has its problems. They sometimes pay consultants good money for advice. I shall consider myself repaid if a few administrators of technical aid give serious attention to the experiences related in this case study.

I would like to record here that I have enjoyed a most satisfactory career in the business of foreign aid. Nowhere could I find more dedicated colleagues than my compatriots in AID. I still believe wholeheartedly in the agency's goals. What bothers me most is not the agency itself, but the way it and its employees have been treated by the United States Congress and each incoming administration. Foreign aid has been a political football, and though it's here to stay, its implementing agency has repeatedly been torn asunder. Before it can recover, the process begins all over again.

There is a need for all aid administrators to be taken step by step through the operations of a genuine technical assistance project. An increased understanding and appreciation of the process hopefully will improve their administration in the interest of the taxpayer and those people of developing countries we seek to help. I trust that this case study may help serve that purpose.

All of my colleagues in Indonesia played a part in the case study, but I am particularly indebted to Ignatius Tarwotjo, M. Sc.; Dr. Sugana Tjakrasudjatma; Tito Soegiharto; Djoko Susanto; and Dr. Alfred Sommer; who were my closest associates and good friends. Thanks also to Lestari Kadarisman who typed initial drafts on her own time when she might have preferred a rest, and the final drafts were typed at my Bandung home by the sweetest of all wives, my own Tarinee. Finally, I am thankful to Professor John D. Montgomery of Harvard and Dr. Delbert Myren of the World Bank for their helpful comments on an early draft, to Dr. Marcus Ingle of Practical Concepts Inc. and Professor L. Gray Cowan of State University of New York at Albany for their most helpful hints on improving the presentation, and to Dr. Winfield Niblo, who in the midst of his own restless search for post-AID retirement usefulness volunteered to save me postage by xeroxing the manuscript in Denver and passing copies to interested reviewers and prospective publishers.

Combating Nutritional Blindness in Children

(Pergamon Policy Studies—57)

1 Introduction

This is a case study of the organization and operation of a single international technical assistance project, the Nutritional Blindness Research Project, in Indonesia. The writer sets forth the history of this project with the hope that it will have some influence on the attitudes of aid administrators and serious students of economic and social development administration and international technical assistance.

The author undertakes this task with a background of heavy involvement in technical assistance planning and administration in Washington, D. C.; India; Sri Lanka; East Africa; Vietnam; and Thailand. This experience is derived from over 25 years of employment as an officer of the United States Government in the Economic Cooperation Administration (Marshall Plan), Technical Cooperation Administration (Point IV), Foreign Operations Administration, International Cooperation Administration, and the Agency for International Development.

TECHNICAL ASSISTANCE: REACTIONS

During the period 1951-76, the United States Government Agency for Overseas Technical Assistance not only underwent a change in name, it also was studied and restudied. Its basic legislation was changed a number of times. Its scope and functions were both enlarged and restricted. Its policies and procedures were repeatedly revised. For long periods the agency seemed to be in a condition of perpetual reorganization. Personnel were frustrated by the attention to paperwork often at the expense of performance and achievement. Recipient governments suffered from planning programs on the basis of the latest American aid policy only to have it change the following year.

The author participated in some of these studies and some of these changes. In many respects changes were for the better. However, over the years, it appeared to the author that many people joining the organization were increasingly less vocal about their knowledge of technical assistance (TA) processes than their experience warranted. They appeared more and more to demand a mechanical approach to the planning of technical assistance programs based largely on the application of modern management control techniques and information retrieval systems.

There is no doubt that such techniques are quite useful in modern organizations and there is no doubt that they can be used to advantage in certain aspects of foreign aid programs, including technical assistance, if applied correctly. But to consider the wholesale application of these techniques to the detailed planning of hundreds of TA projects around the developing world betrays a gross misunderstanding of the complexities of technical assistance.

TECHNICAL ASSISTANCE: THE PROCESS

In its simplest terms technical assistance is a process of one individual or organization helping another individual or organization to solve a problem. Presumably the assisting individual or organization possesses some special knowledge or experience in greater degree than the recipient of the aid, and that greater knowledge or experience is expected to have a beneficial result in solving the problem at hand.

Technical assistance takes place within the whole spectrum of human activity: agriculture, nutrition, health, population, public administration, transportation and communication, education, housing, urban affairs, etc. It can involve the drafting of legislation and the developing of an organization to foster the growth of farmers' cooperatives or trade unions. It may be applied to the renovation of school curricula and the development of text books more appropriately suited to the state of technology in the particular country. It may involve a bold new experiment in developing health delivery services in poor rural areas using medical technologists, better trained midwives, low paid volunteers, and a referral service rather than attempting the impossible task of training sufficient physicians to remain in the villages. It may involve temporary consulting work or long-range institution building. It may involve a single advisor, a consulting firm, or a team of university professors and researchers.

Technical assistance today is the main business of a whole range of international organizations as well as an instrument of foreign policy for a number of governments in developed countries. Many American universities, consulting firms, and voluntary organizations are engaged in the process, often obtaining grants or contracts from the United States Agency for International Development (USAID) or international organizations to partially or wholly finance their undertakings. Most often the technical assistance is provided to or through an agency of a national government in the developing world.

Technical assistance projects are not trouble free. Perhaps more often than not, unforeseen problems arise which alter the nature, required resources, and scheduling of the project.

Building a bridge is a complex affair, as is sending a man to the moon, but within a certain degree of definitude, the engineering elements of such a project can be planned in fairly minute detail from beginning to end with a foreknowledge of the materials, equipment, and skills needed at each stage. The project goes forward with a single controlling manager or coordinator, and where the concerned individuals and support systems behave in logical, predictable fashion, it proceeds with great precision. Technical assistance most often is not like that; it is a sensitive process, manipulated by fallible human beings within the context of different cultural systems, political systems, and administrative structures, all leading to a degree of uncertainty.

Donors and Recipients

In a technical assistance project, the recipient agency is of utmost importance. Some of the manuals of technical assistance planners in donor agencies betray their insensitivity to this fact. They seem to assume that a project is managed by the donor and scheduled in accordance with its appropriation cycle. However, the recipient agency frequently puts as much or more resources into the project than the donor, almost always has a larger stake in the project, or should have, and definitely undergoes the larger risk.

Technical assistance involves a problem in cross-cultural communications. No matter how educated and Westernized the recipient country's personnel appear, they still possess a set of fundamental beliefs and views of life which are grounded in their culture and which differ from the ways Americans look at things. It is easy for some Americans to discount this factor, particularly if most conversations are with other Americans or with local employees who have learned how to cope with their foreign bosses. An occasional chat with civil servants of the national government may not serve to change their minds. This situation is different for Americans engaged for long periods in technical assistance projects who work constantly in a problem-solving context with members of the other culture. The experience can be rewarding, but there still is a communications problem which is not simply one of language difference.

The American aid agency has its decision makers: a Congress which sometimes denies the funds requested, and a new administrator or new mission director who wants to change existing policies and programs and impose his own system of priorities. The agency undertaking a TA project, whether a university or voluntary agency, has its review boards and headquarters administrators who determine what the agency does and how its employees go about performing its tasks.

The recipient government also has its decision makers; it experiences cabinet changes, and has a parliament with members who seek votes in their home constituencies, a bureau of the budget, a civil service system, and its own appropriation cycle. Its leaders sometimes revise their policies and priorities, and the administrative structure may be a wonderful mystery to the outsider.

When these systems confront each other in a technical assistance project, plans are sometimes revised. <u>It is the author's experience that good technical assistance planning must assume that changes in plans will become necessary as the project proceeds</u>. (1) Projects should be planned to achieve the projects' goals. However, those plans should call for periodic review by the various parties concerned of where they are, what they have achieved, what problems need to be solved, and where they should go from the present situation. This calls for a maximum delegation of authority by the administrators at the donor's headquarters to their agents close to the scene of action. It also requires a great deal of patience and understanding at donor headquarters.

INDONESIAN PROJECT

This project focuses on vitamin A deficiency as a causal agent in childhood eye disease. This comprehensive and action-oriented research project aimed at achieving quantitative increases in knowledge about such eye disease. The Indonesian Government has given high priority to completion of the project so that it can use the findings for programs in the third five-year plan beginning in 1979. Aid agencies, such as the World Health Organization (WHO), United Nations Childrens

Fund (UNICEF), and United States Agency for International Development (USAID) consider its completion to be of importance because the methodology developed, the experience gained and the new knowledge obtained will be useful elsewhere in the developing world. These interests coincide with objectives of the American Foundation for the Overseas Blind (renamed Helen Keller International on January 1, 1977) which instigated the project as a means of obtaining more precise information needed to reduce world blindness.

The difficulties encountered in the organization and staffing of this project are similar to those met in numerous undertakings elsewhere in the developing world. Being a relatively short-term undertaking, however, it did not offer the long-term employment incentives inherent in an institution building project. Indonesian approaches discussed later in this case study, suggest that such problems can be resolved where there is sufficient will.

The project is a complex one in the important roles played by a large number and variety of participating organizations, both Indonesian and international. While the project is a creature of the Indonesian Ministry of Health, its participants report to the minister through different channels, and the relationships of these participants to one another are critical to the efficient operation of the project. In addition to the American Foundation for Overseas Blind (AFOB), external contributors include the World Health Organization (WHO) and UNICEF, as well as two branches of USAID.

As might be expected, the budgetary practices and funding procedures of these organizations had an impact upon the conduct of the project. Equipment deliveries could be critical, and planned lead times were sometimes insufficient. Frequently ad hoc approaches were needed to overcome interim difficulties.

Helen Keller International (HKI) assigned two American personnel to the project, Dr. Alfred Sommer as research science advisor and the author as administrative liaison officer. Both had extensive experience in the developing world, but as students of technical assistance are aware, each new experience can be a unique one.

XEROPHTHALMIA: AN INTERNATIONAL PROBLEM

> Xerophthalmia...has been recorded in early writings... for example, Eber's Papyrus, an ancient Egyptian medical treatise of about 1500 B.C., recommends ox liver or the liver of a cock as a curative agent. (2)

When I began this case study, prevalent wisdom produced estimates of 16 million totally blind people in the world. (3) Xerophthalmia (blindness due to a nutritional lack of Vitamin A) was considered a threat to one million children in the developing world each year, of whom 100, 000 became blind annually and an equal number died, most under six years of age.

These estimates seemed bad enough. However, the World Health Organization has now revised them upwards to 40 million blind people. (4) This situation is expected to worsen in the developing world as populations increase. Sir John Wilson, Director of the Royal Commonwealth Society for the Blind, believes that "the number of blind could double by the end of this century." (5) UNICEF offices in Asia estimate that there are now 300, 000 blind children in Indonesia, at least 250, 000 in India, and 200, 000 in Bangladesh. (6) Moreover, the First Assembly of the International Agency for the Prevention of Blindness at a meeting in Oxford in July 1978 suggested that at least a quarter of a million children are likely to suffer blinding xerophthalmia annually. (7)

Xerophthalmia

Xerophthalmia is a progressive disease caused by a diet deficient in vitamin A (avitaminosis A), and occurs most frequently in association with protein-energy malnutrition. It adversely affects the eyes, internally by lowering the sensitivity of the retina to light, and externally by disrupting the epithelia of the cornea and conjunctiva. It seems to be more widespread and serious in the rice eating countries of Southeast Asia than in other regions of the world. (8) Xerophthalmia generally occurs among poor people who cannot afford meat, milk, eggs, and fruits; among uneducated or isolated people who are unaccustomed to eating leafy green and yellow vegetables; and among those who do not understand the connections between the food they eat and their ability to see. "Rarely is a case found among middle income or rich children." (9)

Vitamin A deficiency not only causes blindness, but an international task force considered it to be "a problem with undesirable consequences to health, such as inadequate growth and development and decreased resistance to infection, as well as ocular lesions (xerophthalmia) and blindness. (10)

Xerophthalmia is preventable and to a certain extent reversible. Caught in time, before its blinding stage, called keratomalacia, the effects of most of the other stages, such as night blindness, conjunctival xerosis, Bitot's spots, and corneal xerosis, can be reversed, and the patient's vision restored to normal or with only partial impairment. Additional reasons for attention to the disease include the suggestion that the very existence of xerophthalmia in a given population represents widespread subclinical forms of vitamin A deficiency.

> The population "at risk" may be many times greater than the population evidencing xerophthalmia. If a population is "at risk" with respect to vitamin A then stress factors, such as infectious diseases or seasonal food shortages, assume special significance. (11)

HELEN KELLER INTERNATIONAL

As of January 1, 1977 Helen Keller International (HKI) became the new name for an old voluntary organization, the American Foundation for the Overseas Blind (AFOB). Since the technical assistance agreement with Indonesia was signed before the change in name, however, the AFOB designation was used in Indonesia throughout the project. For many years it supplied books and other study materials printed in Braille in many languages, helped establish learning and training centers, and provided other assistance around the world aimed at educating and rehabilitating the blind. In 1971 the organization decided to step beyond its traditional role of helping people already blind and to become actively engaged in the prevention of blindness as well.

In past efforts HKI depended primarily upon contributions and bequests from the American public. However, international recognition of the vitamin A deficiency problem and its susceptibility to prevention led to the availability of grants and contracts from international aid agencies, such as the United States Agency for International Development (AID), WHO, and UNICEF. Similarly, these agencies and others, such as various Lions Clubs around the world, have supplied assistance directly to projects also assisted by HKI and sometimes provide funds to HKI to carry out activities developed and proposed by HKI.

International efforts to reduce vitamin A deficiency were given additional impetus by United States Secretary of State Kissinger's remarks at the World Food Conference in 1974. During the following year an AID-sponsored ad hoc group formed the International Vitamin A Consultative Group (IVACG). Membership is composed essentially of scientists and officials from WHO, UNICEF, AID, HKI, the Royal Commonwealth Society for the Blind, the International Association for

Prevention of Blindness, the United Nations Food and Agriculture Organization (FAO), the Pan American Health Organization (PAHO), and other bilateral organizations. The group has been meeting annually to provide guidance on (a) needed research and field programs, (b) possibilities of joint funding for major programs, and (c) needed workshops and seminars. The intent of this international coordinating activity is to minimize duplication of research, encourage execution of major projects beyond the financial scope of any one organization, and ensure dissemination of information and new knowledge to concerned organizations and individuals. (12)

HKI has assisted governments in conducting national assessments and surveys and advised on mass distribution of vitamin A capsules, nutrition education, and food fortification. Its activities have been global, including assistance to El Salvador, Haiti, Afghanistan, the Philippines, Bangladesh, and Indonesia. The most ambitious vitamin A research effort to date is the project in Indonesia where clinical experience and survey findings are aimed at the planning of practical programs to reduce the incidence of xerophthalmia.

> ...the prevention is more important than the cure. We cannot contribute more richly to the service of mankind than by protecting sight. (13)

2 Development of a Research Project

DEVELOPMENT

> Our conclusion...is that planning...requires a set of complementary roles--initiators (idea people), influentials (to support a proposal), brokers (who gain support or effect compromises among various formal organizations), and transmitters (government officials and others who make final decisions). This scheme suggests a series of practitioner roles (or roles and resources of others) that a planning organization needs to command in order to be effective. (1)

Xerophthalmia has received attention in Indonesia for decades by many investigators. Some consider that the true public health weight of the problem in Indonesia is obscured because its victims often die before they can be reported as blind.

In 1973-75 the government of Indonesia carried out a pilot program to distribute massive doses of vitamin A in capsules to every preschool child in 20 selected subdistricts on the island of Java, simultaneously conducting an evaluation assisted by HKI (then AFOB). Basic concerns were the efficiency of the delivery system and the effectiveness of the semiannual capsule in reducing the incidence of xerophthalmia. The evaluation raised wholly new questions, however, as to the nature and cause of the blinding aspects of xerophthalmia, especially the relationship of infectious disease and the impact of socioeconomic and environmental factors. (2)

In November 1974, WHO and USAID convened a meeting in Jakarta on vitamin A deficiency and xerophthalmia at the invitation of the government of Indonesia. The meeting reviewed priorities for research and action programs. It specifically recommended research related to (a) clinical, biochemical, and dietary methods for assessing vitamin A status; (b) epidemiology and prevalence of xerophthalmia; and (c) action programs. (3)

Indonesian ophthalmologists and nutritionists keenly interested in developing future action programs attended the meeting in force. A number of other countries were represented by prominent scientists involved in vitamin A and xerophthalmia. Among the participants were Dr. Susan T. Pettiss, HKI Director of Blindness Prevention, and Dr. Alfred Sommer, a young American ophthalmologist/epidemiologist from the Wilmer Institute of Johns Hopkins University. The latter had already served as an AFOB consultant on vitamin A deficiency surveys in Haiti and El Salvador and possessed distinct ideas about the kinds of research results needed for the planning of action programs. Some of the Indonesians present requested of Dr. Pettiss that HKI provide advice on future programs and involve Dr. Sommer if possible.

Later, back in the United States, HKI asked Dr. Sommer to design a research program which would elicit the kinds of clinical and socioeconomic information needed for action programs. Dr. Sommer was convinced that Indonesia was the most logical site for conducting such research, and HKI sent him there in the summer of 1975 to do a feasibility study. The first two weeks were spent in meeting with Indonesian scientists and officials to discuss their respective ideas on the subject. In the company of several Indonesians, he traveled around Indonesia for a month, examining facilities and clinical records, and finding out what kinds of people would be available for the research. A week was then spent in writing the proposal which was reviewed with the Indonesians and Dr. Pettiss who had flown in from New York. The proposal was then rewritten. At this point it was generally assumed by all concerned that HKI would employ Dr. Sommer to help the Indonesians carry out the proposed research.

In subsequent months the budget was reworked via correspondence between Indonesia and New York, and HKI officially presented a proposal to AID for substantial financial support of the project. The original contract was signed on May 28, 1976 and amended on September 30. Under this contract AID agreed to provide about $1 million toward HKI costs of helping the Indonesian government carry out the research.

This contract was sponsored by the Office of Nutrition, Technical Assistance Bureau (TAB) of the AID headquarters in Washington rather than with the local USAID mission in Jakarta, because TAB was concerned with research that had worldwide implications. TAB, however, had no direct connection with the government of Indonesia, and had no way of verifying Indonesian arrangements for the project except through the USAID mission in Jakarta. On the other hand, the Indonesian government needed assurance of AID support before it could sign an agreement with HKI.

It usually takes more than the agreement of technically interested people to initiate an international technical assistance project. In this case an official agreement could be reached only after all concerned parties had been involved and provided clearance. The Indonesian Cabinet Secretariat had to give its approval. The planning body (BAPPENAS) had to be assured that the project was in line with government plans and that budgetary needs were met. The governor of West Java had to approve project activity in his area. These clearances could not be obtained prior to the initial contract signing in Washington in May. As a result the date which appears on the official HKI Indonesian government agreement is August 30, 1976 (see Appendix I). Dr. Sommer arrived in time to sign the agreement on behalf of HKI.

If USAID and Jakarta had been responsible for this project, it would not have obligated American government funds until all arrangements had been cleared by the Indonesian government, as it would have obligated the funds by intergovernmental agreement. AID in Washington had obligated the funds by a contract with HKI which required the latter to perform a job to get reimbursed. To do the job, HKI had to assure that the Indonesian government participated. In achieving these assurances, the local USAID provided valuable assistance.

THE PROPOSAL: A SHORT DESCRIPTION

According to its AID contract, HKI was to conduct a program in Indonesia the purpose of which was:

> (1) To evaluate a methodology for establishing the magnitude and geographic distribution of vitamin A deficiency related corneal destruction; (2) to define, epidemiologically, xerophthalmia of varying degree of severity and severe keratomalacia in order to identify the factors responsible for the occurrence which are amenable to effective intervention; and (3) to develop a methodology to utilize these findings in the design of national intervention programs.

This contract between AFOB (HKI) and the Agency for International Development was signed May 28, 1976. It provided for a planning and preparatory phase to be completed by December 31, 1976, during which the contractor would prepare detailed work plans, recruit and train staff, mobilize equipment, and prepare citizen groups to be included in subsequent activities. Phase II was to begin in January 1977 and run approximately two years during which the following four interrelated studies would be conducted:

1. A study of 5,000 children between 6 and 60 months of age to determine the incidence of each stage of severity of xerophthalmia and the epidemiologic characteristics thereof.
2. A detailed clinical, biochemical, bacteriological, and epidemiological investigation of clinical and hospital patients presenting vitamin-A-deficiency-related corneal disease, together with detailed information regarding their responses to alternative treatment regimens.
3. An evaluation of the effectiveness of bimonthly distribution of massive doses of vitamin A supplementation to preschool children in reducing keratomalacia and testing the feasibility of using village level lay workers in such a distribution program.
4. A countrywide prevalence survey to evaluate a methodology and determine the magnitude and geographical variation of the problem.

The contract also provided for a Phase III during the final months of the project for analysis and reporting.

It was planned from the outset that the project would be headquartered at the Cicendo Eye Hospital in Bandung, the provincial capital of West Java located 180 km from Jakarta. The Cicendo Hospital is probably the most active eye hospital in the country and has the largest xerophthalmia caseload. Its director, Professor T. Sugana, had a strong public health and field orientation and had demonstrated strong interest in xerophthalmia. Cicendo already contained a small bacteriology and chemistry laboratory and served as the eye training center for nurses throughout Java. Last but not least, it had space which could be converted into offices for headquarters personnel and a ward and clinic in which to center Study II activities.

While Cicendo seemed the most ideal location for housing headquarters and Study II activities, its location in Bandung offered several other advantages. One was the historical record of a high concentration of xerophthalmia cases within a two to three hour drive from the city (see Table 2.1). It was suspected that other surrounding areas not using the reporting clinic also would prove to have a high prevalence of the disease, would be less "contaminated" by ongoing modernization activities, and thereby offer a potentially ideal site for carrying out Studies I and III.

Table 2.1. New Cases of Xerophthalmia (X) at Selected Eye Hospitals, 1974

Location	Hospital	Total Cases of X	Cases of X Types 2 and 3 (Corneal)
West Java			
Bandung	Cicendo	387	164
Cikampek	Cikampek (clinic)	312	113
Central Java			
Jogyakarta	Dr. Yap	55	21
	Gajah Mada	120	111
Demarang	Dr. Karyadi	324	(?)
East Java			
Surabaya	Undaan	171	40*
	Dr. Sutomo	No data	

*includes pure conjunctival xerosis

Source: "A Proposal for the Characterization of Vitamin A Deficiency and Xerophthalmia in Indonesia, A Basis for the Design of Effective Intervention Programs," (Prepared for the Ministry of Health, Government of Indonesia and the American Foundation for the Overseas Blind, revised April 1976).

Among Bandung's other advantages were the presence of the Institute of Technology of Bandung (ITB) with its data processing facilities and the Pasteur Institute with its facilities for bacteriologic support. Moreover, in comparison with other possible locations in Indonesia, Bandung was only a three hour drive from Bogor, where serum for vitamin A levels spun and frozen at Cicendo could be transported to laboratory facilities at the Nutrition Institute for analysis, and only a four hour drive from Jakarta, location of the Ministry of Health, USAID, UNICEF, WHO, the international port and airport, and Customs.

The above description is drawn largely from a revision of the original proposal dated April 1976. (4) This revision contained a work schedule which was already out of date, but reflected the initial scheduling of the Indonesian planners and their American consultant. The initial schedule was contained in the Indonesian budget presentation for the Project (see Figure 2. 1).

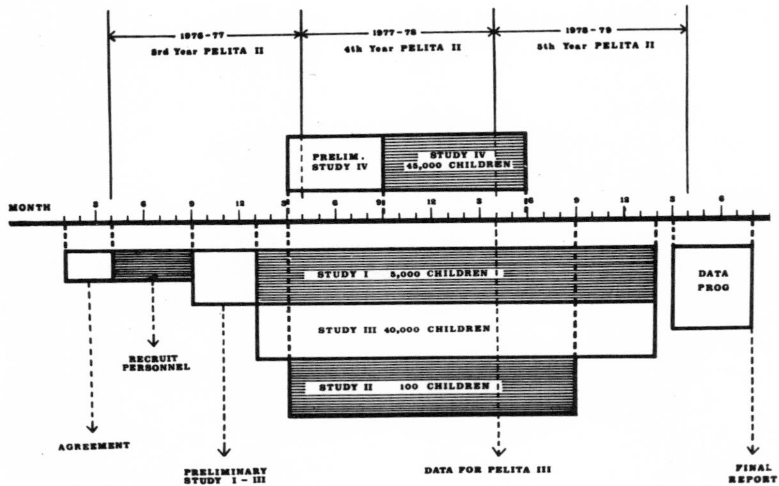

Fig. 2. 1. Initial work schedule. (Note: the references to PELITA II are to the Government of Indonesia's second five year plan. The third five year plan begins in fiscal year 1979-1980.) (5)

Source: See note 4.

What were the chances of this project succeeding? At this point it may be useful to quote briefly from reviews of the proposal undertaken by the Vision Research Committee of the United States National Eye Institute at the National Institute of Health.

> The time proposed for these studies (I and IV) appears very tight - no provisions have been made for emergencies or other possible delays. Can one realistically expect to maintain the proposed schedule?
>
> Although the principal investigator has had considerable experience in epidemiology and work in developing countries, he appears to be somewhat unrealistic in his approach to a long-term study

using primarily the technical people in the host country. From experience of other workers with the surveys conducted in developing countries, it is apparent that in long-term studies there is a high turnover of native personnel which often causes serious problems in terms of replacement and in maintaining an on-going program. This could be a serious deterrent in the present proposals where standardization of eye examinations by field personnel could make or break the validity of the survey.

This is an ambitious program that probably will not accomplish the stated goals. It should, however, provide information on the effectiveness of vitamin A supplement and help resolve questions of extreme importance due to the prevalence of destructive corneal disease in developing countries.

The original proposal mentioned several events which would present time constraints on the project. Two of these need to be mentioned: (a) preparations for national elections in early 1977, and (b) the changing dietary patterns of the people during Ramadan Id, particularly in 1977. However, the time required for Indonesia clearances of the Indonesian/HKI agreement presented the first real time constraint. As seen in Figure 2.1, it was hoped that recruitment for the project could begin in April 1976 after signing of the agreement in the first quarter of the calendar year. With signing of the agreement on August 30, it became necessary to organize, recruit, and perform preliminary work on Studies I, II, and III simultaneously during the final four months of 1976 if field work actually was to begin in January 1977.

3 Initial Organization and Staffing

> The rational tradition generally assumes that once the best alternatives (policies and projects) are identified and planned, implementation will proceed. This is rarely the case. (1)

What were the staffing requirements of a comprehensive research project such as this? The initial budgets indicated the staffing requirements envisioned by the project planners.

Study I required a team of 16 persons including an ophthalmologist, pediatrician, nutritionist, supervisory nurse, five nurses, an enumerator, two census workers (7 months only), two aides, and two drivers. Study II was originally envisaged as a part-time job for a team of 11 persons including an ophthalmologist, pediatrician, nutritionist, four eye nurses, a hospital nurse, a driver, and two aides. Study III required a team of 31 persons including an ophthalmologist, eye nurse, three supervisory nurses, four census workers (4 months only), an enumerator, a driver, and 20 local aides (who would begin 4 months after the others). Study IV required three teams. Each would comprise 11 persons consisting of an ophthalmologist, supervisory nurse, nutritionist, six enumerators, an aide, and a local person who would help make arrangements to ease the work of the team.

To provide direction and support to these four studies, which embraced a total of 6 teams and 91 persons, the planners envisaged a small headquarters or general support staff of 17 individuals comprising the project manager, clinical investigator, administrator, finance officer, supply officer, statistician, 2 statistical clerks, 3 drivers, 3 aides, and 3 secretaries. Overall policy direction would be provided by the director of the National Institute for Health Research in Jakarta who would spend one-sixth time on the project.

Shortages of Trained Personnel

> Severe shortages of trained planners, administrators and technicians plague nearly every Third World country. (2)

In a country where trained manpower is in short supply, it may seem surprising that the responsible government officers conceived of this large, scientific project as a practical possibility. What incentives could be offered to attract highly qualified individuals away from other positions in order to accept jobs which would last only two to two-and-a-half years, or would the government force responsible people out of their current positions in order to perform the temporary, high priority tasks of this research project?

The answer is that for most professional people the government simply added tasks from the research project to their already existing responsibilities. Thus the project manager, "Pak" Tarwotjo, also happened to be head of the Ministry of Health's Nutrition Academy in Jakarta. He also had major responsibility for a large nutrition loan made by the World Bank. Tarwotjo, understandably enough, found it necessary to travel a large part of the time; yet he found it possible to be in Bandung three days most weeks, sometimes more.

To provide adequate assurance that key individuals like Tarwotjo were able to devote sufficient time to the project, the budgets provided for an incentive scheme. The government could provide a per diem allowance for a maximum of 18 days per month from which the individual would pay his travel and other expenses. In addition, the project offered incentive pay which was substantial when compared with the base salary received from the government. For those persons newly hired by the project, i.e. those persons who had no base salary from a permanent government institution, the project paid the entire salary. In addition, the physicians were provided extra payments to compensate for their loss of private practice while participating in the project.

These additional payments were outside the government's budget and, therefore, budgeted by HKI and presented to AID in the original project proposal. This point will be discussed in the budget portion of

Chapter 7 but here the initial organization and staffing of the project will be discussed.

The selection of Ignatius Tarwotjo as research manager seemed assured many months before the project started. He was well-known to HKI as principal evaluator in the earlier evaluation project. While there were problems in his selection because of his other substantial responsibilities, there were also certain merits. His professional background, proven capability, and experience in planning the project were invaluable. Moreover, as head of the Nutritional Academy, he commanded the respect of nutritionists all over the country who had graduated from that institution. Such allegiance was useful, both for employing nutritionists by the project and for obtaining the cooperation of nutritionists and other health officers in the various provinces where the project required administrative liaison and help.

The choice of Dr. Sugana Tjakrasudjatma as clinical investigator was also an excellent one. As director of the largest eye hospital in the country, he commanded the respect of ophthalmologists and the medical profession in general. In July 1976 he informed HKI by letter that the hospital had vacated the rooms needed for project offices and that four nurses were available. At a later stage, it will be seen that he played a unique role in getting Study II started.

Tarwotjo needed a couple of deputies to help him manage the project. Despite his standing in the Department of Health, it was obviously not possible for him to spend too much time fighting the budgetary and administrative battles of the project, and he needed some help. As head of the Nutrition Academy, he did not enjoy ready access to the budgetary and bureaucratic mysteries of those parts of the department which furnished funds for the project, i.e., the National Institute for Health Research and Development and the Directorate General of Community Health. Tarwotjo succeeded in recruiting two persons who helped fill the need. One was Tito Soegiharto of the Nutrition Directorate, part of the Directorate General of Community Health. Tito was chosen as project administrator. The other was Djoko Susanto, statistician at the Nutrition Research and Development Center at Bogor, which administratively reports to the National Institute of Health Research and Development. He was chosen as project statistician.

HKI located an American in Jakarta to help with administrative matters. He represented HKI in discussions with Indonesia government ministries and USAID and worked on visa and other administrative matters for the incoming project scientist. The finance officer from HKI headquarters in New York visited Indonesia during August, set up bank accounts in Jakarta and Bandung, set up a bookkeeping system for handling HKI funds, and interviewed a prospective project finance officer who expected to retire shortly from an Indonesian government position.

By the time the American project scientist appeared on the scene in late August, however, prospects for project success had taken a turn for the worse. Not only was the Indonesian government-HKI Agreement not yet signed, but AID was threatening to withdraw its support if it were not signed quickly. Tito Soegiharto had been hospitalized by an auto accident; Dr. Sugana had been hospitalized with a back problem, which would keep him out of action for a prolonged period; the locally recruited liaison officer was seeking another job; and Tarwotjo met the project scientist with the news that other work pressures prevented him from participating in the project. Last but not least, the project possessed no desks, chairs, telephones, vehicles, typewriters, or typists. At this point, a decision had to be made whether or not to proceed with the project. Was it worth the effort? Could it be done?

The completion of government clearances for signing of the agreement was probably the decisive factor. After signing the agreement, Dr. Sommer proceeded to Bandung with Tito Soegiharto, who had just gotten out of the hospital, and with a promise by Tarwotjo that he would visit Bandung within a month.

Dr. Sugana was available for valuable bedside consultation during the first few months and gradually regained his strength and became ambulatory. However, it appeared that the project would never get off the ground within existing government administrative restrictions. During the first month of frustrating attempts to work within the system, several significant events took place. The first was a visit to Bandung by Tarwotjo and the chief of the Nutrition Directorate of the Department of Health in Jakarta which led to some favorable decisions. The second was a meeting in Jakarta with the official head of the project, Professor J. Sulianti Sarosa, Director of the National Institute of Health Research and Development, who had been out of the country since the arrival of the project scientist. A key decision at this meeting was to set up a project steering committee with the following membership:

Chairman	Professor J. Sulianti Sarosa, M.D., Ph.D. Director, National Institute of Health Research and Development, Jakarta
Vice Chairman	S. Malasan, M.D., M.P.H. Chief, Nutrition Directorate, Jakarta

Advisor	R. Soebekti, M.D., M.P.H. Director General, Community Health, Jakarta
Secretary	Ignatius Tarwotjo, M.Sc. Head, Nutrition Academy, Jakarta
Members	Sugana Tjakrasudjatma, M.D. Director, Cicendo Eye Hospital, Bandung
	Uton Mochtar Refei, M.D., M.P.H. Health Inspector, West Java Province, Bandung
	Darwin Karyadi, M.D., Ph.D. Chief, Nutrition Research and Development Center, Bogor
	M.L. Misbach Staff National Institute of Health Research and Development, Jakarta
Observer	Alfred Sommer, M.D. Project Scientist, Helen Keller International

Professor Sulianti Sarosa, Chairman of the Steering Committee, was well-known nationally and internationally in the field of health and nutrition research. Before she retired in late 1978, she provided leadership, made a number of useful suggestions, and used her prestige to help the project. Reporting to her within the National Institute of Health Research and Development was the chief of the Nutrition Research and Development Center at Bogor, Dr. Darwin Karyadi. Not only was he a well-known nutritionist, but his participation in the steering committee was of value because part of the project budget came from funds under his control. The other part was controlled by chief of the Nutrition Directorate Dr. Malasan, who served as vice chairman of the steering committee. Within the Department of Health, Dr. Malasan reported to Dr. Soebekti, Director General of Community Health, who served as advisor to the steering committee. After it gradually evolved that Tarwotjo could serve as project manager after all, he became a natural secretary for the committee, responsible for arranging meetings, preparing many of the presentations, and carrying out many of the decisions. Participation of Dr. Uton Refei, the West Java health representative, was also of value because his help was necessary in obtaining clearances for project operations in that province. He was always a helpful member of the project and came to its aid on several occasions.

One may wonder that the author considered it important to discuss the establishment of these high level governmental relationships at the outset of the project. The reason lies in experience with projects which encountered difficulties: "The principal barriers to an effective project are not technical but are personal and political." (3)

Initially it appeared that the Nutrition Research and Development Center in Bogor could not release Djoko, project statistician, to work in Bandung and that the statistical staff would have to be located at Bogor. As this would have created very difficult logistical problems, the decision to relocate Djoko in Bandung was a welcome one. Because of Dr. Sugana's illness, the project hired the Study I ophthalmologist several months prior to the anticipated requirement. Participating in detailed planning for Study I operations and training of nurses and enumerators, he also made the necessary preliminary arrangements with local government entities. His early recruitment was one of the first extra-budgetary burdens to be experienced by HKI.

The initial group responding to the advertisement for nurses and enumerators was clearly unqualified and had to be turned away. From a second group, 25 were selected for training. During initial training their salaries were reduced, so the total matched the amount budgeted for the purpose. The training included interview techniques and the recognition of ocular disease. Final selection was based on their performance in a written exam and field exercise and their fluency in Sundanese, the language prevalent in the area chosen for Study I operations. At this point three nursing academy graduates were hired as supervisory nurses, and twelve high school graduates were hired as nurse-enumerators. This group continued to train in the hospital and classroom for an additional month.

The finance officer retired from his government position, set up his accounts, and reviewed them with Price Waterhouse officers in Jakarta. Another retired government officer was hired as supply officer. Three secretaries were hired. Desks and typewriters were procured. Negotiations with various agencies of the Ministry of Health, the West Java Government, UNICEF, and USAID resulted in the loan to the project of a Jeep and Volkswagen Safari from the West Java representative of the Health Ministry, a Land Rover from UNICEF, and three rather used Holden station wagons from USAID. Despite initial frustrations, it was clear that a great deal of momentum had been created. The project was now underway.

4 Study I: Periodic Observation of the Children at Home

...it is important for studies to be made at different seasons. (1)

Project managers are constantly making decisions, either using already developed standards or criteria for making those decisions or developing their own criteria based on their knowledge and experience, perhaps tempered by some kind of international or locally acceptable standard. Frequently, we find that a research or survey team has to develop new sets of standards and criteria, sometimes from scratch. It is possible that case studies like this can perform a service in relating how previous project managers have tackled problems in the past, thus easing problems for future project managers. In time, perhaps, some standardized approaches can be developed, particularly for those kind of efforts which are repetitive and occur in many if not most technical assistance projects. The preparation of surveys would seem to fall in that category.

During early October 1976 the American scientist, the project statistician, and the Study I ophthalmologist began planning the subsequent field work of Study I. The general area of operations had already been selected, an area near the town of Purwakarta. It was now necessary to select the actual study sites. For the purposes of Study I, it was preferable that the sites chosen contain a high evidence of disease and a "virgin" population uninfluenced by recent government development activity. To make this selection it was necessary to do the following:

1. Identify villages with high referral rates to the Cikampek Eye Clinic and the Community Health Center at Plered.
2. Identify nearby villages with very low referral rates; generally these villages were less accessible by major roads

or public transport.
3. Conduct minisurveys in both types of villages to determine which low referral areas had the highest prevalence of disease, and how these virgin areas compared to the high referral areas.

To accomplish the first two purposes the ophthalmologist and statistician reviewed all xerophthalmia records at Cikampek and Plered for the years 1972-76. They confirmed or rejected the diagnosis on the basis of the clinical description, the patient's age, sex, and village. They calculated population figures for each year on the basis of official estimates for 1976, and established referral rates for each village.

After mapping this data, the team chose a number of villages in which they conducted one-day prevalence surveys. The final site selections were based on the following criteria:

1. A high incidence of disease as estimated by the minisurveys.
2. Low clinic referral rates.
3. Sufficient population to provide the necessary number of children (five to eight thousand) for the longitudinal field study.
4. Accessibility to facilitate field work.
5. Absence of government plans for significant development projects over the next two to three years.
6. Absence of other field survey work in the area.
7. Dietary patterns representative of most of Java (primarily rice consumption).
8. Cooperation from local officials.

Related activity was the preparation of forms for the first step of Study I, the survey and census of families for over 5,000 children under six years of age to obtain baseline economic and social data prior to actual clinical examinations. These forms were devised jointly by Tarwotjo, Djoko, and Sommer after consultation with Indonesian survey specialists in village areas. They were field tested during the minisurveys by the enumerator trainees and reviewed by computer specialists at the Institute of Technology in Bandung. English translations of the two basic interview forms, the family baseline data form 103A and the individual baseline data form 103B, are found in Appendices II and III.

When dealing with rural people who have little education and income, it is often difficult to determine whether respondents are answering truthfully and accurately regarding questions of wealth and income in monetary terms. They probably don't really know how to answer such questions, because they most probably built their own homes and largely subsist on crops they produce. It is sometimes more practical to deal with matters which can be visually checked by the enumerator. For these reasons, Study I did not attempt to obtain wealth and income data in monetary terms. Instead, the forms asked for information on land and livestock owned, the materials used in constructing the family house, the source of drinking water and lighting if any, the occupations of family members, years of education, the basic foods eaten, and whether they were homegrown or purchased from the market. Ages of family members were based on the Arabic calendar and converted to the international calendar by the enumerators.

Of course manuals for these forms had to be written, as well as general operating instructions for the survey teams in the field. A number of auxiliary forms also had to be devised. These included a family census form which would register each family member and summarize results of repeat examinations to be held over the next two years. Each family was to retain a registration form which could be checked by the enumerator on repeat visits (see Appendix IV).

OFFICIAL COOPERATION

Governmental approval and complete understanding of projects and related responsibilities is necessary to avoid the experience encountered in Ecuador.

> The Ecuadorean Government officials, from the Minister down, misunderstood the purposes of the project and their responsibilities under it. We should have made these more clear. (2)

The remaining principal activity was the soliciting of official approvals for field work and visits to local government officials and village leaders to explain the project and get their cooperation. Though the project had a letter of approval from the Ministry of Health, it was also necessary to obtain clearance for field work at every administrative level. The importance of treating this matter seriously cannot be overstated. The district and village heads could be helpful to the project only if they were fully knowledgeable about its importance and benefits; failure to obtain local government clearance can result in difficulties.

This latter point was exemplified when the project earlier sent the nurse-enumerator trainees into a rural area for field exercises. The responsible officer attempted to shortcut the clearance process.

He selected an area where a group of university students had already been cleared for survey work with the thought that it was a simple addition which would not require clearance. This was a mistake. The field exercise had to be postponed until clearances were obtained. On the other hand, officials who became knowledgeable about the project complained when the minisurveys resulted in decisions to eliminate their areas from Study I.

At this point there arose a slight technicality in the contract between HKI and AID. The contract contained the following stipulation:

> At an appropriate time during the first phase (planning and preparation) and before the second phase of the study can begin, the project will be reviewed by AID and the Host Government and concurrence by both on plans and preparations for work must be obtained before the second phase can be implemented. The results of Phase I will be submitted in sufficient time to allow required reviews and approval prior to January 14, 1977.

HKI headquarters in New York informed the project scientist on November 3 that an AID representative and a team of consultants were planning a site visit between January 25 and February 1. The project scientist prepared an interim report dated November 19, which he submitted to HKI and the Indonesian government. On that day the project steering committee met to discuss the report. Suggestions were made and problems were discussed, but no questions were raised about the move into the field. After modification to reflect these discussions, HKI submitted the report to AID in Washington.

It is generally a good idea when undertaking a large, comprehensive project to pause for a moment at some stage and review progress and plans with knowledgeable colleagues. It is a good idea to conduct an evaluation of a project in midstream. Without such evaluation it is not unusual to report satisfactory progress until the last steps of a project, at which point schedule delays and additional costs are brought to attention. It is probably not a good idea, however, to stipulate that a project come to a halt until a review is completed, particularly when faced with the problems of communicating between Bandung, Jakarta, New York, and Washington and the logistics of putting a team of consultants together from four American institutions to travel to Bandung for such a review. And who represented AID in this case? The consultants on the spot? AID in Washington, which would provide written concurrence after receiving a report from its consultants? This was not clear.

The review team report is dated January 1977. However, the team left Jakarta for the United States on January 31, the project received copies in March, and never received word as to any AID decision. At it turned out, the team apparently interpreted the census and survey as part of the planning and preparation stage, because they referred to the beginning of "full field operations about March 1." (3) Meanwhile, the census and survey work began in the field on January 3, 1977.

THE CENSUS SURVEY

> ...planners seem to systematically underestimate the difficulties of data collection. (4)

The census survey had two basic purposes. The first was to find and register in Study I children under six years of age who would be examined repeatedly by a clinical team over the next two years. The other was to obtain comprehensive data on the social and economic status of the families of these children, which would be correlated later with the presence or absence of eye disease caused by vitamin A deficiency.

Census Survey Procedure

For purposes of the survey the enumerators were divided into three groups, each headed by a supervisory nurse. Each numerator was given a team number which appeared on every form for which he was responsible. The entire group was put under the charge of the Study I nutritionist who reported to the project statistician.

During the survey, the enumerators, nurses, and nutritionist made their homes in the villages where they worked, using their per diem to rent rooms and purchase food from the villagers. During the day they went from house to house seeking families that contained one or more children less than six years of age. They numbered each house and family and tacked an identifying sign on each house. They patiently interviewed senior members of each family, visually checking where possible the data they were given. At night they met together to check their forms, relate the problems encountered during the day, and how they solved them.

Difficulties Encountered

Family registration form.

One problem was the color of the family registration form to be retained by the families. While foreign advisors should check out their survey forms with knowledgeable local people, doing so does not always guarantee their utility. In this case, Indonesians decided on the pink color of the registration form which some Indonesian families were reluctant to retain because to them it represented communism. Luckily, enumerators were able to persuade the villagers that the pink color did not represent communism. They pointed out that the national flag was in fact red and white.

For most of January the teams stayed in the field, working Saturdays and Sundays in order to complete the survey more quickly to get a longer vacation period prior to beginning the base line clinical examinations. During the first crucial weeks of the survey, the project statistician lived and worked with the enumerators so he could understand their problems and advise them. Subsequently, he spent more time in Bandung where he hired a statistical staff to check forms and perform calculations. Completed forms and maps collected at least once weekly were doublechecked at project headquarters by the statistician's staff. Feedback of results to the enumerators served to correct and improve their work.

Errors commonly made at the beginning of the survey were easy to spot because of cross-checks built into the forms. Form 103B, for example, asks for the birth date of the child and its age in completed months and years. At the beginning, enumerators registered the age as one year even though the age in months was eleven or less. On noting this phenomenon, an American staff member discussed it with the project statistician. It turned out that the latter had already met with the nurses and enumerators on this very point. At the end he became so overwhelmed by their arguments that he became convinced, as they were, that no child could be less than one year of age. This, of course, is a common view of age in a number of Asian countries. However, once the forms were made up, it was important that everyone agree to the meaning of each question and the related instruction.

A little carelessness was also evident in the initial weeks of the survey. In filling out the forms, the enumerators usually started with the head of the household, identifying him as number 01. They then identified his wife as number 02, and so on. Form 103B requested the identifying number of the family member who takes care of the child. The practice referred to above led some of the enumerators to write 02 without stopping to think. Persons in Bandung doublechecking these forms sometimes had reason to question this number, because the household might contain several mothers of children under six. Sometimes the person caring for the child was also head of the household, having been divorced, separated, or widowed. In a family of two, the number 02 referred to the young child itself.

In Bandung the clerical staff transferred the name, age, and sex of each family member to a Census Book, Form 106 (see Appendix V). Copies of this form were given later to the clinical team to help identify children registered in the study and to record the results of subsequent examinations. One column was reserved for the identification numbers of persons taking care of each child under six. At the beginning, clerical staff considered it less troublesome to just write "Ibu" (Indonesian for "mother") in this column. Since the grandmother or an older sibling often assumed prime responsibility for the child, this practice also had to be stopped. Gradually, both the enumerators and the statistical clerks became a seasoned team.

Housing.

Initial plans called for the Study I nurses and enumerators to remain in the villages during the entire study period of 1978-79. After completion of the census survey, they would periodically examine the children and be checked by the ophthalmologist and pediatrician, with the latter two also responsible for less frequent comprehensive examinations. This plan was dropped for a couple of reasons. For one thing, as noted previously, only three of the field staff hired turned out to be real nurses and qualified to perform physical examinations. Most compelling, however, was the loss in weight and deterioration in health experienced by the nurses and enumerators during the months of village living while carrying out the census survey. They apparently were unable to continue a heavy workload on a villager's diet. The whole team, therefore, was given a week off in early February. These events necessitated a change in plans to include setting up a field headquarters and living quarters for the Study I team. The project leased a large house in Purwakarta in February for this purpose.

During the same period project staff completed development of forms for the base line clinical examinations, wrote a manual to cover operational procedures, purchased some equipment and supplies, and planned other details. At this point it was decided that one team of enumerators would remain in the villages until May to complete the census survey. The other two teams were joined by the ophthalmologist, pediatrician, and nutritionist to form the Study I Clinical Team. After a short period of training, the team moved to Purwakarta in mid-March. Its members pooled their per diem to pay the largest portion of the house rent; HKI put up the balance, another previously unbudgeted sum.

Elections.

Over the horizon for some months had been lurking a troublesome problem which began to loom larger and larger. Could project work in rural areas continue during election campaigning? By late January it was learned that the campaign period would last from February 24 to May 1. The government issued an order which permitted basic research to continue if crucial to fulfilling the objectives of REPELITA II and REPELITA III, but prohibited all research with social and political implications.

This prohibition was understandable in the Indonesian context. Political activities in the past had been particularly volatile in the countryside. The widespread turmoil of the late Sukarno era had climaxed in extensive deaths in 1966-67 in the wake of a communist-inspired insurrection which threatened the nation's existence. Since that time, the government had pursued a policy of stabilization and development, legally restricting the number of political parties, and the nature of their activity while giving voters a chance, first in 1971 and again in 1977, to voice their political preferences.

No matter how sophisticated Westerners view such matters, in the context of the Indonesian countryside it was natural to view the Study I team as a vehicle of the government party. It was necessary to obtain a clarification of the government's attitude toward the project. With gratification project officers received a Minister of Interior letter saying he had no objection to continuing the project and that he deferred to the government of West Java for a decision. Subsequently the governor signed a letter saying he had no objections, but leaving the final decision to the local authorities, which meant the regent (Bupati) of Purwakarta Regency (Kabupaten).

The Bupati held a meeting of local government staff, including representatives of the military forces. The meeting ended in a deadlock. It was going to be difficult for the Bupati to make a final decision. At this point, Professor J. Sulianti Sarosa, project director, chairman of the project steering committee, and director of the National Institute of Health Research and Development, took an active hand by signing a letter "for the Minister" in which she stated that the project was a very important one for the government. The Bupati acted on this letter in mid February, deciding that project work could continue except on the actual days assigned to each party for political activity. Since there were four parties, this meant four days in each village. Since different days were assigned in different villages, the team had no difficulty in scheduling its work to avoid villages where campaign activity was being conducted.

Workload.

By the end of February an unforeseen problem arose. The three statistical clerks had fallen far behind in the checking of census forms and the transfer of data. In March the clinical team would begin its work with a mammoth set of additional forms to be checked and data to be transferred. It was important that initial errors be checked immediately so the team would not perpetuate those errors. The original budget had provided for two statistical clerks, but the three currently employed in that capacity could not keep up with the workload. Project officers located three recent high school graduates expecting to go on to higher education or accept permanent positions elsewhere at a later date. In the interim period they were willing to accept temporary positions at a low salary, Rp. 30,000 (about ($75.00) a month. They went quietly to work and gradually caught up with the backlog. Study I could proceed to the next phase.

CLINICAL EXAMINATIONS

On March 14, 1977 the clinical team, comprised of the ophthalmologist/team leader, a pediatrician, a nutritionist, two nurses, eight enumerators, and two drivers, moved with their equipment into the field headquarters house in Purwakarta. The next morning they began work at the first field site, accompanied by the research manager, statistician and the two Americans on the project. Also present for the first couple of days was Dr. Muhilal, a biochemist from the Nutrition Research and Development Center in Bogor, who provided guidance in drawing, spinning, and storage of blood samples drawn for laboratory analysis.

The first day the team returned to headquarters early, having examined only 60 children. They used the rest of that day to review experiences and to plan procedural improvements for the next day. The two Americans returned to Bandung at the end of the second day. However, the principal scientist had to return to the field the following day to substitute for the ophthalmologist whose wife was reported to be having a baby at the hospital. It turned out to be false labor.

The changes in Study I procedures created a need for two four-wheel drive vehicles rather than one because the whole team moved with its equipment to a new study site each day. Often, even these vehicles were unable to reach the study site. In many cases the team had to walk long distances; in a couple of cases they had to hire boats. By the end of May the rainy season came to an end, which made for somewhat easier, though often dusty walking conditions.

Examination Procedure

Four days of the week the team examined children. They were soon able to examine more than 100 per day. On Friday mornings the team went to Bandung with the forms completed that week, listened to problems raised by clerical checking of their forms from the previous week, ordered medical supplies and forms needed the following week, and met with the project's executive staff to discuss problems and obtain guidance. They sometimes also brought in patients for treatment at the Cicendo Eye Hospital. Later, those involving active corneal disease were referred to the new special Study II clinic.

Upon arriving at a study site, the team generally stopped first at a central point (CP) previously selected in discussions with the local people. Usually this was a house donated for the day, though sometimes it was a school or village office. A portion of the team would remain there to prepare the work space. Sometimes part of the work had to be performed outdoors, which was satisfactory if it was not raining or the sun shining too brightly. Chairs and tables always seemed to be available. The scales were usually hung from the eaves of a building or from a nearby tree.

The enumerators set out with their maps, census books, and forms on which they had already filled in family and individual identity information. At each house the enumerator conducted a short interview, largely on a medical history of the children, and obtained information on new family members and those who died or left the family since the census survey. Before leaving the house, the enumerator encouraged the parents to bring all children under six to the CP.

In most study sites the response was excellent. Many individuals seemed to consider the examination to be a special affair. Mothers dressed themselves and their children in their finest and brightest clothes to join the growing throng at the CP. Frequently, fathers and older siblings came along to help with the small children. On the whole, those people at home when the enumerators visited agreed to bring their children to the CP. The team found through experience that calling on rural homes around noon achieved the best attendance of children at the CP. They therefore revised their work schedule to arrive at the homes at that time.

The doctors had to confirm on a clinical basis the ages of children already recorded in the study. Visiting the CPs from time to time, the author was bemused by the friendly arguments with the parents who usually knew the Arabic month in which the child was born, but often had difficulty in remembering the year. During the census, the enumerators had tried to relate a child's age to some well-known event. Evidently this scheme had not been entirely successful, so the project devised forms on which it would report age changes to the computer facilities at ITB.

The clinical team examined the children for height and weight, eye problems, and general health, including nutritional status. If a child was ill, the doctors would treat him and refer him to the appropriate medical authorities. Children with active, curable eye disease were referred to the Cicendo Hospital and taken there in a project vehicle.

For every child diagnosed as abnormal in his eye exam, the nurses took a pinprick blood sample from the child's finger, and the nutritionist conducted a special dietary interview which included a review of the child's food consumption over the past 24 hours. The doctors also identified a matched control to compare with each child diagnosed as abnormal. The child identified as a control was the next child examined who was of the same age and sex as the diseased child. Toward the end of the day, it was sometimes necessary to detail previously examined patients in order to assure selection of matched controls. Parents of control children were then encouraged to have their blood examined and to provide dietary information.

Initially, the ophthalmologist alerted other team members to the presence of diseased children and controls by marking both forms with a red "X". When some villagers complained about the communist connotation, the ophthalmologist quickly exchanged his red pencil for a blue one.

It was fun to watch the antics of the children at the CP. A few were apathetic, most at least slightly uneasy, some suspicious, and there were those who were frightened to tears. The good-natured ophthalmologist joked with the mothers and bantered with the children, but if a child put up a fight, the doctor grasped him firmly, placed his head on his lap, pried his eyes open, and the project had its data.

The pediatrician sometimes had greater problems because he had to probe the child's body with his hands, and worse yet with a metal instrument Westerners know familiarly as a stethoscope. Moreover, most of the children were scared to death of being placed in the scale or against the wall for measuring height. Rarely a boy would break away and make a run for it. The older children, the laughing onlookers, would go after him and carry or drag him back from the mud or gravel where he had thrown himself head first.

Before providing the census books to the clinical team, the project's statistical group identified certain families as random samples for the initial clinical round. Every tenth family was identified to provide dietary information. While interviewing the families at home, the enumerators took additional time to secure this information for the random sample family as a whole and for each of its children under the age of six. Every twentieth family was identified to provide children for the blood examination. Thus, the project was able to secure information from which it could compare data on diseased children and controls with a random sample of the population. The random sample list was revised on each subsequent clinical round.

Blood Tests

Blood samples were taken to the Purwakarta field headquarters each night where the blood was spun and frozen. After the team delivered the blood at Cicendo on Friday mornings, it was taken to the nutrition laboratories in Bogor, usually by the project statistician when he returned to his base position at the Nutrition Institute on Friday afternoon. Technicians at Bogor then analyzed the blood for its vitamin A and carotene content, retinal binding protein, albumin, and prealbumin.

The blood examinations entailed some difficulties. First, the project had to procure a small refrigerator for the field headquarters. Then as the team began to experience frequent failures in electrical supply, the project procured a small standby generator. More importantly, the mothers did not understand the importance of having their children's fingers pricked for blood if their children appeared healthy, as did many of the matched controls and random samples. As a matter of policy the team exhorted but did not insist on blood examinations, particularly for children under one year of age.

Community Liaisons

> To the extent that members of a target group are suspicious of an agency, communications channels will be blocked. In such a situation a 'multi-purpose worker' will be necessary. His main job will be to establish linkages between the organization and the target group. As these linkages are established, it becomes possible to reintroduce specialists, now trading on the 'multi-purpose workers' relations. (5)

A special problem arose in several neighborhoods of one village where many parents failed to bring their children to the CP. In one neighborhood the refusal rate was 70%, in another 100%. The ophthalmologist reported that the people of the area openly spoke of the project as a "blood sucking" project, and that a local religious teacher (ajengan) had taken the children into his school and kept them there while the team was in the vicinity.

The neighborhood (kampung) of 100% refusal was accepted as a special challenge. The kampung was quite isolated from outside activity, was quite poor, and traditional in its outlook. Project analysts suspected generally that such populations were especially susceptible to xerophthalmia.

Just prior to this incident, the project had hired a teacher of social work, Achlis, on a parttime basis. He was asked to look into the incident and advise. On Tuesday, July 18, 1977 Achlis visited the Camat (head of the kecamatan, also known as subregency or subdistrict), as well as an influential modern minded religious leader of the area. The Camat reacted seriously to the information provided by Achlis and tended to blame the village head (the Lurah) who continued to be actively engaged in private business and neglected his official duties.

The Camat related that the isolated people of the area were greatly influenced by the ajengan, who owned a mosque and religious school. During the past village elections the ajengan had supported the present Lurah in his candidacy, but since then they had had a falling out. The Camat was uncertain whether this fact or the ajengan's opposition to blood samples was the more important cause of the team's problems. In any case, the Camat decided to send a letter to the Lurah instructing him to give his personal attention to the problem.

Achlis also visited the Lurah, who stated he had been in Bandung during the team's visit to the kampung. He considered this a very difficult kampung in tax matters. However, he thought the team's problems were normal and caused by the children's fears of vaccinations and blood-taking. To improve community relations he was giving village finances to construct a mosque owned by the ajengan. Achlis had performed his function well, having followed the Rothman study's injunction that linking agents should take advantage of local opinion leaders in conducting their work. (6)

The next day the Camat took his police commander, the Lurah, and the influential, modern minded religious leader to the kampung where he hoped to meet the ajengan. The ajengan was not at home, so the Camat used the ajengan's house to meet with citizens of the kampung. Here the earlier project briefings of local government officials had positive results.

The Camat explained the functions of blood in human life, and why it was necessary to examine the children's blood. The citizens then informed him of rumors which had arisen before the arrival of the clinical team. People of a neighboring kampung had said the clinical team was taking large quantities of blood, enough from each child to fill a large bottle. The Camat explained that the team really only drew a pinprick of blood from a child's finger, a much smaller amount than was usually taken from hospital patients. Indeed, the team carried bottles containing cough syrup, similar to blood in color. They gave this medicine to children with coughs. The Camat asked whether it was true that ajengan had taken the children into the school to guard them against activities of the clinical team. One elderly man sharply contradicted this notion, referring to it as slander. According to him, the children had simply run away screaming and hid themselves.

The Camat then decided to hold another meeting at the ajengan's mosque on Friday after noon prayers. At that meeting, the kampung residents agreed to cooperate with the clinical team, but requested that it not come during Ramadan, the Muslim fasting month, and that mothers be permitted to hold their children when blood was drawn.

It was important, of course, that the linking agent, Achlis, not only influence local groups to make use of existing services, but that he also influence a modification of policies and practices of the service organization so as to be more in tune with client needs and aspirations. The Study I team took Achlis' advice, returned to this kampung, and completed its examinations in early August 1977, prior to the beginning of Ramadan. This kampung was one of the last study sites visited during the first round. The team was given a week's rest before beginning the second round. They had examined 8,700 children in the first round, more than had been required for Study I.

Subsequent Examinations

The project reduced its coverage during the second round, and the team completed its reexamination of about 5,000 children in November. One disturbing thing occurred; two children free of eye disease during the base line clinical round were now totally blind. They were sent to Cicendo for treatment with the hope that vision would be partially restored. Obviously, vitamin A deficiency can have quick devastating effects.

During the third and fourth rounds, fewer children were available for examination. Records showed predominant causes were not migration and noncooperation. For the most part, it appeared that the mothers had taken their children with them to the rice fields. Perhaps periodic visits by the clinical team were getting a bit stale. On the other hand, the ophthalmologist reported that the women lost Rupiah 150 (about 35¢) a day if they stayed at home, particularly during planting and harvesting seasons when plenty of work was available.

The absences were particularly troublesome because they usually occurred in areas which earlier recorded the most disease, the poorer areas where no doubt the families needed to earn as much money as possible. Moreover, the team recorded a decline in the rate of disease, reflecting the possibility that the children with the disease were the very ones who did not appear for examination, and during the season when previous investigations had indicated that the disease occurred most frequently and seriously. How could the project accurately record seasonal variations under conditions like this?

Incentives for Participating Families

In the early days of Study I, project officers had considered passing out incentives to participating families. They decided not to do so on the original clinical round because of possible accusations of bribery during the election campaign. However, the team had passed out cough syrup or medicine for diarrhea and skin rashes when needed. On the second round, they distributed cheap spools of thread, but the ophthalmologist reported the mothers showed little interest in this gift.

During a meeting in March 1978, project leaders decided they would experiment with incentive payments during round five beginning the following month. About a week prior to the clinical team's visit to a kampung, a messenger would spread the word of the impending visit and that Rupiah 150 (about 35¢) would be available for every mother who brought all of her children to the CP.

5 Studies II and III: Children in the Hospital—Study and Treatment

THE PLANNING PHASE

With Study I proceeding well, project personnel were able to turn their attention to other matters. April and May of 1977 were spent largely in detailed planning for Studies II and IV. During the first half of May the project scientist was out of the country, mainly to attend the International Vitamin A Consultative Group meeting in Basel, Switzerland.

By late April the planners decided they must begin Study II by June 1, although the equipment had not yet arrived. The director of the Cicendo Eye Hospital made available two large adjoining rooms for the study, one for a special children's ward and the other as a clinic. During late April and May these rooms were completely renovated, and necessary equipment, medicines, and other supplies were purchased and placed in readiness for the study to begin.

A small administrative and budgetary problem arose at this stage. Technical assistance practitioners are painfully aware that seemingly small administrative problems are often more important obstacles to project implementation than the serious technical problems.

Department of Health planners had somehow neglected to budget for use of the hospital space, but perhaps they knew what they were doing. They had also appointed as clinical investigator of the project Cicendo's director, Dr. Sugana, who by now had dispensed with his ambulatory aide and was even taking field trips.

As director of the Cicendo Eye Hospital, Dr. Sugana could not ignore the budgetary problem. As clinical investigator, however, he recognized that a solution was necessary. He sat down at his desk and pondered the problem. Slowly the solution came to him, and he rose to the occasion.

First, he wrote a letter from the clinical investigator to the director of the Cicendo Eye Hospital. His letter described the needs of the hospital director to make the necessary space available. After receiving this letter, Dr. Sugana read it carefully and composed his reply. He said he recognized the importance of the project to eye health in Indonesia, he appreciated the requirement for hospital space, and therefore, he was responding to the clinical investigator's request by making two rooms available to the project free of charge.

The Study II ophthalmologist and pediatrician had been identified previously. The ophthalmologist, Dr. Nani Emran, was a staff member at the Cicendo. The pediatrician, Dr. Tien Tamba, had been running the malnutrition ward for children at the Hasan Sadikin Hospital in Bandung. Both physicians retained their former positions, but spent most of their time working on Study II. They participated in developing forms for Study II and spent two days in the field observing the Study I clinical team before opening the Study II clinic.

It will be recalled from Chapter 4 that a nurse and five enumerators had been left in a village to complete the base line census and survey for Study I. They completed this work in late April, had a week's vacation, then went into training for Study II. This included a week on the job with the Study I clinical team and two weeks at the malnutrition ward at Hasan Sadikin where they learned to care for children, take various blood samples, and prepare milk.

There was some difficulty in obtaining a full-time nutritionist for the study. Initially, the West Java Health Service made two nutritionists available for in-service training with the Study I clinical team. At first, project officers thought they were to make a choice. Later it turned out that the nutrition unit of the West Java Health Service could not make either person available full time and was only considering the loan of one or perhaps two persons part time, but this was impractical. The project then located a nutritionist who was not available until September. However, his wife was also a nutritionist. Though out of practice for several years, she was available for the interim period.

As indicated in Figure 2.1, the original time frame for Study II was 19 months. Initial plans were to study 100 children during that period, with the staff working part time. However, the doctors were available to work full time. Moreover, Cicendo Hospital referrals of xerophthalmia cases to the project scientist in recent months were more than past records had led project planners to anticipate. It now seemed important that the project not turn away any cases. Each needed immediate treatment and was potentially important in learning more about the etiology of xerophthalmia and the phases which lead to keratomalacia and blindness. Thus, project officers estimated they could study at least 100 children within a 12 month time frame and decided to do so.

Related to this decision was the status of Study III. As recalled from Chapter 2, Study III was planned as an evaluation of the effectiveness of a bimonthly distribution of massive supplementary doses of vitamin A to preschool children to try to reduce keratomalacia. As originally planned, this intervention trial required a population of 40,000 children randomly allocated, half of whom would receive vitamin A and the other half placebos. This calculation was based on an estimated prevalence of keratomalacia of one per thousand children and an incidence of at least twice this.

The minisurveys, however, indicated that the purportedly high prevalence areas actually yielded lesser prevalence rates. This, coupled with the large fluctuations in annual referral rates to the eye clinics in the area, led the staff to reconsider this complex approach to intervention trials. Other concerns included the logistical problems of vitamin A and placebo distribution by village personnel, the dangers of mixups despite supervision, and the difficulties of assuring that the capsules were actually used. These concerns raised doubts about the feasibility of executing such a large study with success. On the other hand, with a lower rate of keratomalacia than anticipated and with the biases of hidden noncompliance and a probable attrition through dropouts, a much larger trial would have to be mounted which, under the circumstances, was unfeasible (the Site Visit Team reported on this in its "Review of Government of Indonesia and American Foundation for Overseas Blind Project," January 1977).

By January 1977 the project staff had modified these plans -- an interim decision as it turned out -- to provide for a therapeutic trial of vitamin A in conjunctival disease and nutritional deficiency in a population of 3,000 children enrolled by the census and mapping techniques of Study I. The Study I group went ahead to census and actually examine 8,700 children which would have given this interim plan a head start.

As detailed techniques were developed for conducting Study II, however, it became apparent that identical information could be obtained with less manpower and vehicle requirements by attaching Study III to Study II. These techniques will be described later in this chapter.

STUDYING AND TREATING THE DISEASE

Study II

The children for Study II came from the following referral sources:

1. Xerophthalmia cases entering Cicendo and the Hasan Sadikin Hospital in Bandung. There were referred to the Study II Clinic before receiving any therapy. The Hasan Sadikin Hospital also referred non-xerophthalmia malnourished children to Study II to act as matched controls. This latter group turned out to be so small, however, that the study developed other techniques to identify its matched controls.
2. Active corneal disease cases referred from the district hospital in Purwakarta; the clinics in Plered, Cilegong, and Cikampek; and cases identified by the Study I clinical teams.

All children registered in Study II were offered free hospitalization and therapy as well as free room and board for an accompanying adult. Those referred from the clinics, the Purwakarta Hospital, and the Study I team were given free transportation by project vehicles. In addition, if the accompanying adult, usually the mother, was found to be the prime wage earner of the family, she was given Rupiah 150-200 (nearly 50¢) per day toward her family's support. These were important concerns in the Indonesia context, as will be seen later in this chapter. Nevertheless, many parents refused to come to Cicendo or to bring their children.

In fact, only about half of the parents permitted their corneal diseased children to remain in the hospital once they got there. Thus, there was a natural division of study groups: those remaining in the ward who got vitamin A plus a high protein diet, and those not hospitalized who received vitamin A and whose home diet presumably remained unchanged. The nutritionist calculated the dietary intake for all children remaining in the ward. Every attempt was made to keep a child on the ward at least two weeks; some parents insisted on going home earlier, and some stayed longer.

All corneal patients underwent complete ophthalmologic and pediatric examinations. The opthalmologic component included a history of the sickness and previous therapy given, if any, an external examination with handlight, a slit lamp examination with flouroscene, bacteriology where indicated, vital staining, a Schirmer test, dilation, a night blindness test in a darkroom, and indirect ophthalmoscopy for retinal lesions and status of the disc. In selected cases where the child had already lost sight, there was macrophotography and a conjunctival biopsy. The pediatric component included measurement of height, weight, and arm circumference and a tuberculosis skin test. When indicated, a chest x-ray was given at the Hasan Sadikin Hospital. Blood was drawn on all children and analyzed for serum vitamin A, retina binding protein, albumin, prealbumin, and measles titer. The nutritionist collected dietary data on all participants, and a nurse-enumerator recorded socioeconomic data on their families.

For treatment purposes, the first 40 patients were systematically divided into two groups. On the day of admission the first group received an injection of 100,000 international units (IU) of vitamin A, the other group a single capsule containing 200,000 IU. Occasionally, children not doing well on the one-dose schedule received a second dose after two-three weeks. However, because one child demonstrated clearing of corneal xerosis by two weeks and a subsequent relapse in the third week, the schedule was changed with each group getting a second, oral dose of 200,000 IU the second day.

In addition, children who required it received appropriate antibiotics. Those with evidence of systemic illness were treated accordingly, despite the resultant confusion of analysis regarding the effects of therapy on the eye.

All hospitalized children and as many as possible of those not hospitalized underwent daily follow-up ophthalmologic and pediatric examinations. These continued until the lesions completely cleared. Thereafter, they received weekly or monthly examinations. After the first 30 children experienced rather slow healing of lesions, the once daily slit lamp examinations were decreased to twice or three times a week until healing, and subsequently to one on each follow-up visit to the clinic. Any time a patient missed a follow-up examination, the project subsequently sent a vehicle to transport the parent and child to the hospital. This was frequently necessary, as parents saw no reason to undertake an expensive trip to the hospital once their child recovered.

Twice a week the Study II team went into the field. Each time the area selected was the immediate neighborhood of one of the patients who had returned home after hospital treatment. A week before the visit, the physicians sent a letter to appropriate authorities in the area to be visited. These letters indicated the date of the proposed visit and that a central collection point would be needed near the home of the previously hospitalized case.

On arriving in the patient's neighborhood, the team located the patient's home and proceeded to the central point (CP), where a portion of the team prepared the examination site. Three enumerators simultaneously proceeded in three directions, starting from the house of the index case. At every house they inquired whether there were any children under the age of six. Where there were, they filled out socioeconomic information on the family and encouraged the parents to bring their children to the CP. If no children were present, the enumerators quickly moved to the next house. In this manner, the team examined all children from 15 families, about 25 children, surrounding the house of the index case, including 5 random sample families. The team obtained a blood sample and dietary information on all children in random sample families, the family of the index case, children the same age as the index case, and those with night blindness, conjunctival xerosis, or active keratomalacia.

In addition, the team encouraged parents of two-three children at each site to bring them to Cicendo for two-three days of tests. These children were of the same age and sex and if possible, the same nutritional status as the previously hospitalized index case. These became the "selected" matched controls for the index case.

Families in these areas were very cooperative. Possibly because parents of treated children resided in their midst, they recognized that a problem existed, and readily submitted their children for examination. In fact, sometimes the team was deluged with additional requests for examinations by families or a school in the vicinity. The team performed these extra examinations upon request or referred them to the special children's clinic at Cicendo. Those with corneal disease were enrolled in Study II, those without disease in Study III.

Study III

Study III children comprised those referred to the clinic with vitamin A deficiency but with no corneal involvement. They were examined in the same fashion as Study II, except that normally they were not hospitalized, less blood was drawn, there were no bacteriologic studies, and there were no field visits.

Study III children generally were divided into two groups, one receiving a single capsule labeled A (200,000 IU vitamin A) and the other receiving capsule B (undetectable amount of vitamin A $\pm$ 1,000 IU). After three months all children previously receiving capsule B were given capsule A. In the interim they were watched carefully. Any evidence of corneal involvement triggered immediate hospitalization and treatment.

There were two exceptions to these rules. Very few children entered the clinic who were more than eight years old. Some appeared to have Bitot's spots which were resistant to vitamin A treatment; these were rare cases and required special treatment. Thus, no capsule B was given. Instead, all such children were given capsule A on two successive days. If lesions did not disappear after one month, one eye was biopsied then, and the other at a later date. In addition, beginning in late August 1977, no child with 108° or more of conjunctival xerosis was given capsule B; such children always received capsule A.

Some analyses could not be performed because of the lack of equipment. Up to February 1978, no holo-retina binding protein could be analyzed. The equipment was delivered in October 1977. However, it required the advice of Dr. Glover, an eminent biochemist from Liverpool, before the analysis could begin. Also, just a month before Study II began, the Pasteur Institute (Bio Farma) advised that a laboratory accident had destroyed all of their cell culture lines. Until these could be restored, the project could undertake no viral studies.

PATIENTS AND FAMILIES: SOCIOECONOMIC DATA

> Some segments of the population have historically been more prone to nutrient deficiencies than others. Poverty and malnutrition have been closely related. (1)

Dr. Susan T. Pettiss had spent her career in social work prior to her appointment as HKI Director of Blindness Prevention. When she visited the project in mid-1977, she expressed real concern over the children who for one reason or another could not be cured at Cicendo and returned home blind. Subsequently, she obtained HKI support for the part-time employment of an Indonesian social worker. Achlis was hired to visit the blind child's family and community, look for economic and social problems which might have a bearing on the case, obtain help to alleviate those problems, and provide guidance to the family and community in the rearing and education of the blind child so that he/she might not be shunted aside but grow into a self-sufficient, useful, and productive citizen. It was hoped that the Cicendo Eye Hospital would continue the special children's clinic started under Study II and that local organizations might continue the financing of a social worker.

Reports

Achlis' case reports give some behind-the-scenes flavor to the clinical examinations of Study II. Here are excerpts from a few of the author's translations:

1. From 2:00-11:00 P.M. I was engaged in taking home two patients and their parents. This experience may be useful in planning later trips. Going uphill for six kilometers through the rubber estates of village Karoya, the exhaust and muffler of the Holden station wagon was damaged three times. After the second occurrence, I urged the parents to walk home from there. The children were almost in tears, and the parents refused. When the tail pipe broke for the third time and we were short of gas, we stopped at the rubber estates where we got some gasoline and some mechanical help.

   In leaving that area we realized why the parents were unwilling to walk home when we saw several small tigers crossing the road in front of us. Also, the distance was quite far. I recommend we use a jeep to take patients home.

2. All parents staying in the ward are aware they are responsible for their children's care. However, they continually dwell on their household obligations and responsibilities and are always asking when their children can go home.

3. Three mothers have not been visited by their husbands. They complain that they don't have money to buy their children sweets. The project pays Rupiah 150 a day (about 30¢) to each of these mothers, as they are principal income earners in their families. However, they send all of this money home, leaving nothing for themselves or children.

4. My attempts to persuade parents to bring their children to Cicendo for follow-up examinations reveal some reasons for their reluctance:
   a. Some cannot afford transportation. The nine families I visited this month must spend on the average about Rupiah 1,000 (about $2.50) for a round trip.
   b. Some families have other sick members. The Achmads could not bring Tuti, for example, because her father had been gone for three days to obtain treatment in another village. Meanwhile, Mrs. Achmad was busy with a new baby. Likewise, the Atip family could not bring Ajat because Mr. Atip had been hurt in an auto accident.
   c. In some cases there was no one to take care of other children remaining at home. Sometimes the father worked far from home, and there were several small children to care for. For example, the Tarmidi family

lived about an hour's walk from the nearest road with public transport. Mr. Tarmidi's carpentry work took him from home early every morning, and he returned at night. His wife usually didn't try to go to the city on her own, particularly the week her baby had a fever.

d. Some considered their children were already cured, so why return to Cicendo? For example Mrs. Tarmidi said child, Jaja, was quite well and watched TV at a neighbor's every night until 9:00.

5. Visiting the home of Heri, male, 6 months, I learned he died about a week after returning from Cicendo. In fact, Heri's parents have had three children, and all have died. The first died a few hours after birth. The prolonged illness of a three-year-old brother was the reason Heri's parents requested the latter to be treated as an outpatient. Several days after returning from Cicendo, Heri developed swellings on his hands and feet and died. His brother died a week later.

6. Mrs. Kasmin's husband died three years ago, leaving behind six children. The three eldest children from a previous marriage are now adults and working. Of the three remaining at home, the eldest is a girl of 12. She went to school for three years, but is now helping her mother financially by braiding bamboo hats. She can complete a hat in three days, for which she earns Rupiah 250 (60¢). A nine-year-old son in the first grade of school helps bring in neighbor's goats from the field. Icih, the patient, is about six and almost sightless in both eyes.

Before Icih's illness, Mrs. Kasmin worked in a textile mill at Majalaya earning Rupiah 3,000 (about $7.50) a week when working six hours a day. Sometimes she also worked as a farm laborer in planting and harvesting seasons.

The Kasmin family has their own house made of bamboo measuring about three by five meters. Their kampung (neighborhood) is about 1-1/2 km from Majalaya. It is like an island, situated amid irrigated rice fields. The road is passable only by two-wheel vehicle. Though the neighborhood is small, only several hectares, the houses are crowded together like in a city slum. The residents are mainly farmers, farm laborers, factory workers, and home handicraft workers. Physically able men and women work in the factory and rice fields. Elderly people braid bamboo hats or spin thread at home. A person earns Rupiah 10 (2-1/2¢) for spinning a spool of thread and can usually spin seven spools a day. The cost of public vehicle from Majalaya to Bandung is Rupiah 175 (43¢).

7. Pak Sutiarsa lives in an industrial area about 15 km from Bandung. Thirty-five years old, he has a wife and four children. The patient, a four-year-old boy, was their first son and treated well. Experiencing measles at the age of three, his left eye thereafter became red and swollen. The physician at Sutiarsa's factory said it was trachoma, and his attempts to treat the child were unsuccessful. They also tried traditional medicine. Finally, some months later, they took the child to Cicendo, leaving the other children with the grandmother. At Cicendo the doctors removed the left eye and sent him to another doctor to obtain an artificial eye.

   During July, project doctors held a clinic in Pak Sutiarsa's kampung. Four families were urged to send their children to Cicendo. One of the children has now died.

8. The Mimin and Achmad families live in a kampung about an hour's drive west of Bandung. A teacher at a nearby religious school is reputed to treat and cure eye disease. Both families took their children to this teacher before going to Cicendo.

   Mimin and his wife have four children. Mimin himself is one of eleven children and is blind in one eye. He can read, having been to elementary school but not graduating. He earns his living by selling plastic rope and tablecloths at two different village markets, each two days a week. He sometimes also works in construction.

   To capitalize his plastic business, Mimin got a Rupiah 10,000 ($25.00) loan from a neighbor which he repays in monthly installments. From a day at the market he grosses Rupiah 1-2,000 ($2.50-$5.00), earning a profit of Rupiah 2-300 (50-75¢), sufficient to purchase several liters of rice. He makes weekly trips to a supplier in Bandung where he has good credit.

   On August 4, 1977, I visited the family to urge them to take the child to Cicendo. Pak Mimin happened to be at home. We both sat on the floor. He objected to going on Friday, and I thought his objections were religious. When I suggested Monday, he said he did not have sufficient funds.

To Gardujati by public vehicle is Rupiah 150 (38¢) or Rupiah 300 (75¢) for the round trip. A round trip to Cicendo by tricycle rickshaw is another Rupiah 150 (38¢) or Rupiah 300 (75¢). I suggested that he borrow from a neighbor, and he said he would come if possible.

The Mimin family did not appear at Cicendo on Monday. On Wednesday I again visited their house. When I asked Mrs. Mimin if she could come to Cicendo with me, she answered, "Entah," which has two meanings in the Sunda language: "I don't know" and "Who knows?" She answered all questions in the same manner. In my experience this not only indicated confusion, but also a gentle method of refusal. I then joined Mimin's father who urged that we look for Mimin at the market.

When we arrived at the market, Mimin had just packed his goods to go home. When his father told him why I had come, he appeared embarrassed and said he felt the child was already cured. Nevertheless, he brought his goods to the car, and we proceeded to his house where we picked up his child. According to Mimin, most people of the kampung with eye disease seek help from the kyai (religious teacher) at Buniwangi. The Kyai had prescribed chicken liver and recited incantations or prayers, but Mimin had only been able to buy chicken liver on one occasion.

Later, at Cicendo, Mimin showed me a prescription given him by the physician. How could he possibly pay for it? His wife was also upset. She had brought the child at my suggestion, but not to buy medicine again. It happened to be a prescription for ear medicine not in project stocks, but Mr. Fritz agreed the project could pay for it.

9. While at Mimin's house, we were joined by Mrs. Achmad, a pregnant lady with a letter from the Project doctor. Achmad had 11 children, and his wife was about to deliver another. He had not worked for five years because of an ailment in both legs. Two older daughters were working as farm laborers and sometimes got part-time servant jobs at the neighbors.

Tuti, a girl of two, has had eye disease for a long time, and cannot see at twilight. Achmad has taken Tuti to the Kyai at Buniwangi. He had wanted to take her to Cicendo, but had no funds for the trip.

10. Pak Sar'an, Titi's father, lived on a hillside in Kampung Heulet. During the rains of 1976, a rock slide destroyed 30 homes on that hill. Afraid to remain there during the current rainy season, Sar'an hired a vehicle to bring his dismantled house to its present location in a resettlement kampung where he now resides with other evacuees.

    Pak Sar'an now makes and sells bamboo wicker work. The price of one piece is Rupiah 500-1,000 ($1.25-$2.50), depending on its quality and size. The process takes quite a long time and requires borrowing from the owner of the bamboo grove where he cuts the tree. He repays the loans after making a sale in the city.

    Titi's condition was critical when brought to Cicendo in July 1977. Already unable to open her eyes, treatment did not help. She is blind in both eyes. In looking at the condition of her two younger brothers, I fear they too will suffer nutritional blindness.

11. Rasih, female, three years old, was accompanied by her grandmother and great grandmother when brought to Cicendo in January 1978. Her mother remained at home, expecting another child shortly. The whole family lives together in a kampung in Karawang Regency, an area which has suffered food shortages during the past year or so.

    Rasih's grandmother explained that several weeks before arriving at Cicendo the child had suffered diarrhea. The family took a neighbor's advice, squeezing juice from tamarind leaves which they gave the child to drink. The diarrhea stopped, but her fever remained. Several days later, something began happening to the child's eyes, and shortly thereafter they were completely closed. Upon another suggestion from the neighbor, they pounded cassava leaves and squeezed the juice into the child's eyes. In addition, the grandmother licked the child's eyes with her tongue each morning. According to the neighbor, the saliva of a person just awakened from sleep had curative power.

    One morning the child's eyes appeared much different than before, as if they had exploded outward. Frightened, the grandmother told the girl's father, and they decided to consult the village health worker. The latter urged them to visit the polyclinic at Cikampek. This clinic, which cooperated with the project, sent the child to the Study I team at Purwakarta which sent her to Cicendo. According to the Study II team, the child will probably be blind in both eyes.

6 The Equipment Pipeline

Several disruptions occurred during the course of the project. (1)

The AID-HKI contract budget provided only $39,000 for materials and equipment over the life of the project. HKI sought supplementary resources from other agencies that had indicated an interest in the project during its development stage. While the USAID mission in Jakarta was the most important of these, WHO and UNICEF also contributed in important ways. The UNICEF contribution was straightforward and provided no difficulties. It consisted of the vitamin A capsules and placebos, some Salter scales, and the loan of a Land Rover.

WORLD HEALTH ORGANIZATION (WHO) EQUIPMENT

Initial discussions with USAID in Jakarta regarding the supply of equipment and chemicals for the Bogor nutrition laboratory indicated the probability that most of these materials could be procured most economically from non-American sources. Though AID had liberalized its rules regarding sources of procurement under its loan financing, it had not done so for grant technical assistance. It seemed probable that AID procedures for waiving procurement source requirements would prove time consuming and possibly result in adverse decisions. HKI, therefore, approached WHO for a grant to the Bogor Nutrition Research and Development Center. HKI then assisted with the purchase and shipment of the commodities, most of which came from the United States anyway.

WHO had a long-term interest in vitamin A deficiency and had published one of the more definitive works on the subject as a result of the international meeting it had cosponsored with AID in Jakarta in November 1974. (2) It was appropriate to seek WHO participation in the project, thereby helping to ensure its continued interest on a worldwide basis. In early June 1977 project officers received notification of the first delivery of WHO commodities. It was a small package containing two covered metal trays designed for holding surgical instruments when placed into an autoclave for sterilization. This value was about $200.

CUSTOMS PROCEDURES AND PRACTICES

The HKI liaison officer, the author of this case study, decided to test Customs procedures at Halim International Airport in Jakarta. On June 10, armed with a full four months of Indonesian language training on the job, he entered the premises of the Customs building. He succeeded in finding an officer who told him he must start at the information office of the warehouse located nearby, as he needed a special Customs clearance document (PPUD). While standing at the information window, he was approached by a well-dressed Indonesian who asked if he could help. After ascertaining the problem, the Indonesian guided the liaison officer to a building about one km distant where they approached an elderly man seated behind a desk on a veranda in the rear of the building. The liaison officer left his documents with this man, who said he would have the PPUD prepared by 2 P.M.

When returning that afternoon, the liaison officer noted that his Indonesian "helper" had also returned. After the former paid Rupiah 3,000 ($7.50) for the PPUD, the latter guided him to a small office just outside the main entrance to Halim. This office belonged to a private firm with an apparent monopoly on preparing papers for customs clearance. Officers there wanted Rupiah 15,000 ($42) for this service. The liaison officer refused, but after considerable argument and haggling, agreed to pay Rupiah 10,000 ($25.00), and was asked to return the following afternoon. After the liaison officer and his "helper" left the office, the latter asked for Rupiah 20,000 ($50.00) to help with custom clearances. Though he lowered his offer to Rupiah 10,000 $25.00), the liaison officer refused to pay and dismissed him. The next afternoon the liaison officer returned; the papers had been completed, but the boss had left for the day.

On Saturday, June 11, the liaison officer sought out Tito Soegiharto, project administrative officer, who had returned to Jakarta for the weekend. They met at 9:00 A.M. at the Bureau of Logistics, Department of Health. The head of that bureau showed Fritz, the liaison officer, a schedule of legitimate payments to be made at Halim for various services. The minimum cost, Rupiah 15,000 ($42) was what Fritz earlier had refused to pay. Tito and Fritz proceeded to the small office outside of Halim, where the latter paid Rupiah 10,000 ($25.00) and picked up a folder containing all of the documents needed by Customs. Once again Fritz entered the Customs building, this time accompanied by Tito.

On the whole, Customs officials were quite polite, and frequently pushed Fritz to the head of the line. However, there were many officers to be seen, some several times, and procedures were extremely cumbersome. Most officers kept a log in which they entered the case. One put checkmarks beside each of the items listed on the airway bill. Another added them on an adding machine. Some checked the various documents for numbers of copies and others for consistency. Soon all the documents and the folder were covered with stamped dates, titles, and signatures. Sometimes an officer wanted additional copies of a document, in which case Tito left the building to obtain xerox copies. One female officer had to be visited three times. She was so nasty to Tito on the first visit that he refused to return. She scolded him for bringing along a foreigner; she couldn't accept bribes witnessed by a foreigner.

By one o'clock Tito and Fritz completed their tour of Customs, or so they thought. At the warehouse, Cardig Air would not release the commodities because Customs had kept their copy of the airway bill. Quickly returning to Customs, Tito and Fritz persuaded reluctant officers to extract the paper from a filing cabinet already locked for the weekend. By this time, however, Cardig Air was closing for the day and refused to assist further. Fritz returned to Bandung.

Tito returned to the fray Monday. Failing to get the equipment, he passed the remaining documents to Tarwotjo who took them to Bandung. On Tuesday Tito flew to the Outer Islands to begin a three-week series of visits to various provinces to make the preliminary arrangements necessary for Study IV.

Ten days later, Fritz returned to the warehouse at Halim. He was directed to a Customs office in the warehouse, where officers insisted the goods had not yet arrived. In the process of the argument, Fritz discovered that a small slip of paper was missing from his documents. This paper had been signed by a warehouse clerk and given to him nearly two weeks earlier. Either it was taken from Tito during the latter's interim visit, or it was lost. Fritz then went directly to the head of the section and reminded him in Indonesian of their meeting two weeks earlier. The latter confirmed this fact and asked an officer to help Fritz. By this time Fritz decided to hire a "helper," a young man who requested only Rupiah 3,000 ($9.50). He soon introduced Fritz to a smiling, young Customs officer. The helper said this officer could be very helpful if Fritz paid him Rupiah 2,000 ($5.00). The day was getting hotter; Fritz summoned up all the Indonesian language he could muster and spoke in a loud voice, "Why is it that when I am trying to help the sick children of Indonesia Indonesian Customs officers want me to pay for it?"

Many other visitors were trying to get their own goods out of Customs. These onlookers smiled and nodded knowingly. Customs officers appeared embarrassed. One, however, whispered that Fritz should not talk like that; there were many signatures to be gotten, and the officer could be helpful. Fritz was shown the box which was then opened. A small flurry of excitement arose when the Customs official noted three pieces of equipment rather than two. A small spatula had been included in the package. The official then asked Fritz to describe the use of the equipment, which was done. The box was then re-closed and left for Fritz to collect after final clearances were received.

Fritz and his helper then entered the offices of the Cardig Air Company. As they approached the desk of the officer who was supposed to provide clearance, the latter left his seat and went outside. The helper told Fritz the officer would return if Fritz paid Rupiah 2,000 ($5.00). Fritz slipped his helper Rupiah 2,000, and the officer immediately returned.

When they returned to the main Customs building, officials extracted documents from the files and checked them against the forms returned from the warehouse with more stamping, signing, and initialing, and more interviews with Customs officers in the privacy of their offices, finally to return to Cardig Air and the Customs offices near the warehouse where payments were made for storage and handling. At last the ordeal ended, and Fritz picked up the package, paid his helper, and returned to Bandung. The Customs procedures had been tested.

Over the next months Admiral Sudomo, heading a center for law and order, conducted a widespread campaign against illegal payments received by government officials. On September 5, Tito and Fritz were gratified to read an article in the daily Kompas with a picture portraying a confrontation between the Admiral and Mrs. H.S., a Customs official referred to as the "Queen of Graft" at Halim; Tito and Fritz recognized her.

BLOOD TESTING EQUIPMENT FOR VITAMIN A

Measurement of vitamin A in blood is technically more complex than for many other vitamins. Thus one of the critical WHO items was a spectrophotometer required by Dr. Muhilal, biochemist at Bogor. Some of the Study II analyses were impossible without this instrument. The instrument desired was available from the Beckman Corporation in the United States, but not until June 1977. A cable from HKI in New York during mid-August notified the project of its delivery to Halim. A visit to the WHO offices in Jakarta disclosed the existence of documents for several other cartons of chemicals and laboratory equipment which had been delivered at Halim in April. Since there had been a personnel change, no one knew who was to receive these commodities. Muhilal received the chemicals in September and the spectrophotometer in late October. Other WHO-financed laboratory equipment ordered by Dr. Glover of Liverpool was also delivered in late October, just in time to be useful for Dr. Glover's short visit to the project for consultation and training purposes which was scheduled for early November.

Clinical Inconsistencies

These delays in equipment deliveries led to frantic exchanges of cables between Bogor and Liverpool. Finally, Dr. Glover decided to postpone his visit. Unfortunately, he was not available again until February 1978. Meanwhile during November, Dr. Sommer was scanning Study II blood data when he noted some anomalies. According to the data recorded, one patient had an unusually high vitamin A level upon admission. After massive oral doses, the data showed a large decrease. Continuing his investigation, he found additional anomalies. Carefully checking the methods used for drawing and spinning blood and the possibilities of vitamin A contamination in the Study II clinic, he detected a small technical aberration which he corrected. However, he could not account for the inconsistencies between blood results and clinical findings. Looking at results of Study I blood analyses, he found similar inconsistencies in the most recent data.

In early December Dr. Sommer reviewed these inconsistencies with biochemistry staff in Bogor. Subsequently, Dr. Muhilal wrote a technical report which reviewed the possible factors which might influence the vitamin A data. Prominent among these were the decrepit nature of his ancient spectrophotometer and the heavy workload imposed by the project on his laboratory staff. As a result, Dr.

Sommer ordered a drastic reduction in blood drawings for both Studies I and II.

Problems with Scientific Instruments

On December 28, however, a letter from Muhilal stated that his old spectrophotometer was no longer capable of providing accurate vitamin A data. He had been trying to use the new WHO spectrophotometer, but it didn't work either. He attached a copy of the technician's report, which referred to a defective part which had to be replaced. Since such instruments were a rarity in Indonesia, there was no assurance as to when the part could be obtained. One of the instruments ordered by Dr. Glover could be used to obtain indirect readings of vitamin A values, but it wasn't working either. Hopefully, Dr. Glover could get it started after his arrival in February.

During early January 1978, Susan Pettiss again visited from HKI in New York. Fritz and Sommer raised the problem of the spectrophotometer. They could not trust any blood data obtained since the previous July, and now they'd have to await Customs clearance for a replacement part which could fit into anyone's purse. They then remembered that another group of people was coming to Bandung from HKI that month to work on a project relating to education of the blind. Why not have one of them bring the replacement part; why not indeed? Fritz telephoned the Beckman representative in Jakarta and asked him to cable Beckman in California to airmail the part to HKI in New York. He then cabled New York. HKI replied that the last persons coming to Bandung had already left New York before the replacement part was received.

During the second week of February, Dr. Glover arrived in Bogor. On Thursday he and Muhilal appeared in Bandung. Not only had they gotten the new instrument to work, thus providing indirect readings of vitamin A, but even before Dr. Glover's arrival, Muhilal had heroically managed to get his ancient spectrophotometer to produce accurate readings once again.

It was important that all of the blood data be rechecked from July, and it was important that all data were reliable, but Muhilal's lab staff were already tired, and he had a number of other responsibilities. How was the project going to catch up? The only answer was to relieve him of all other responsibilities for several months and to hire at least one additional technician to help him. Muhilal agreed that this could be done, except for one day a week when he had to lecture in Jakarta. His other projects could be turned over to someone else. Sommer agreed that HKI would recompense him for the financial losses he would incur by so doing.

At this point Sommer was off to an international meeting in Switzerland, then on to New York for a conference with the HKI advisory committee. He would return March 1 with the replacement part for the new spectrophotometer. Before departing he asked Muhilal to rearrange his responsibilities with his employer, the director of the Nutrition Research and Development Center.

USAID COMMODITIES

> When voluntary agency executives meet together, it is not uncommon for an agenda of substantive development issues to devolve into discussion of AID bureaucracy and its attendant problems. (3)

USAID in Jakarta was the largest donor of commodities to the project. On June 15, 1976, two and a half months before signing of the HKI - Indonesian government agreement, USAID wrote that it was preparing agreements for project commodities totaling $91,000. At this stage USAID was awaiting assurances from BAPPENAS (the planning agency) that Indonesian government funds were available for the life of the project. Unfortunately, the process had to be started by the Ministry of Health which had not yet written to BAPPENAS. On August 27, the day before the agreement was signed, USAID in Jakarta cabled AID in Washington, D.C. that BAPPENAS had necessary assurances.

USAID in Jakarta specified commodities for the project together with funding citations in a document well-known to AID staffers and called a Project Implement Order/Commodities (PIO/C). In each case the General Services Administration (GSA) of the United States Government was cited as the authorized procurement agent. GSA would then issue purchase orders to the supplier, who would arrange for delivery of commodities to Indonesia. The first PIO/C signed by the director of the Indonesian National Institute for Health Research and Development and issued by USAID on September 28, 1976 covered the procurement of office machines, photographic equipment, and a slit lamp for $14,744, as well as medicinal and pharmaceutical products for $7,305. In both cases someone in USAID had insisted that the commodities be transported by sea. The PIO/C for medicinal and pharmaceutical supplies was amended October 20 with no change in value to authorize air shipment. The PIO/C for office machines was amended the following day to add $1,100 and to authorize air shipment of a portion of the equipment. On October 29, USAID issued a PIO/C for $44,000 to cover the purchase of six jeeps. On January 10, 1977

USAID issued a PIO/C for $8,000 worth of surgical instruments and additional photographic equipment. This document had to be reviewed and approved by AID in Washington and was reissued with no change on April 7. USAID issued a final PIO/C for $2,200 worth of additional office machines and supplies on January 21, 1977.

On the whole these dates appeared to offer sufficient time for delivery of commodities to the project in reasonable fashion. However, as time went by, it became evident that this was not true. The lag between USAID issuance of a PIO/C and GSA issuance of a purchase order seemed particularly unreasonable, and this writer is unable to account for it. GSA issued purchase orders for a few of the pharmaceutical products in January, February, and March 1977. However, most of the items appearing in the September 1976 USAID PIO/C's were not ordered by GSA until May 9, 1977.

The AID on-site review team of January 1977 pointed out the urgent need for expeditious delivery of project equipment, particularly vehicles. Some quotations from their report follow:

> ... some urgent needs exist. Foremost among them is the need for at least 4 four-wheel drive vehicles. If these cannot be provided soon from American sources, tax free purchase from the local market should be most seriously considered. Adequate progress ... is absolutely dependent on frequent access to isolated rural areas ....
>
> The biochemistry laboratory, which is essential to Studies I, II and III, is not yet set up. Every effort should be made to provide this equipment, and necessary supplies as soon as possible, and certainly within the next 2-3 months. Transport by air freight will probably be essential.
>
> Strong efforts should also be made to provide as soon as possible the slit lamp ..., surgical instruments, and other items which are requisite for Study II. Although we are aware of the difficulties and red tape which beset the provision of equipment items for a project of this type, the established and relatively inflexible time frame for this project absolutely requires the availability of all of these items in the very near future. (4)

Officers of USAID in Jakarta reacted sympathetically to the report in varying degrees. The most crucial delay was in the delivery of jeeps. Unfortunately, USAID had been having a problem in clearing its own motor pool vehicles through Indonesian Customs. Influenced by this, USAID had imposed a hold order on the purchase of additional vehicles for Indonesia, including the six for the project which had been specified in the October 1976 PIO/C.

The basic problem was that the Indonesian government for some time had been restricting the entry of vehicles into the country, its objective being to develop progressively their local assembly. In the long run, the government cleared the USAID vehicles. One difference existed, however, between the USAID vehicles and project vehicles. The latter were consigned to the Ministry of Health which had already begun the process of obtaining permits from the various responsible government entities in advance of their delivery.

USAID officers looked into various alternatives for an interim or permanent solution to the problem. Some officers, including a visiting assistant administrator from AID in Washington, thought the situation justified local procurement with AID funds, but this would require a mission request before he could take action. When later approached in Washington, he claimed he had never received such a request. In late March USAID cabled Washington to request that the original order for American jeeps be implemented.

It was during this period of warm discussion that USAID assented to a proposed grant-in-aid of the two well-worn USAID station wagons being used by the project to the West Java health representative in exchange for the loan of two four-wheel drive vehicles. Just prior to this exchange, HKI had expended funds to purchase four new tires. It then sent the four old tires to Jakarta for vulcanizing. USAID also made available an old Jeep Wagoneer. The project, including HKI, spent considerable sums of money over the months on operation and maintenance of these vehicles.

One cause for the radical modification of Study III, as described in Chapter 5, was the shortage of vehicles. Their delivery for Study IV, however, seemed an imperative.

In early development of the project, it was thought that Study IV, the nationwide prevalence survey, could be implemented through the local rental of vehicles and drivers, and original budgets were based upon this assumption. Later, however, it was learned that four-wheel drive vehicles in many places were unavailable for hire. In other places, the cost was two or three times the cost initially assumed. Finally, Indonesian government budgetary rules proved to be a discouraging factor, a topic for discussion in Chapter 7.

Studies I, II, and III managed to progress despite the vehicle and other equipment problems. In August 1977 the project recruited and put into training the 30 physicians and nurse-enumerators required for Study IV. In late August they were conveyed to the field training site in vehicles rented by the project. While training on the job they were transported by a horse and wagon rented by the project. On their return to Bandung, they were conveyed by rented vehicle.

It was understood that the six jeeps were loaded on a ship in Baltimore in late August, too late for the scheduled beginning of Study IV in Bali on October 3. In late September USAID came through with funds for the project to rent vehicles.

EQUIPMENT DELIVERY

There were other causes for delaying delivery of commodities to the project. At an early stage the HKI liaison officer discussed with USAID how he might be kept informed on deliveries of equipment in Indonesia so he could help expedite their delivery to the project. He was told an Indonesian employee routinely notified the Health Ministry, and that in the future he would make copies of such correspondence for Mr. Fritz. This was not done, however.

In June 1977, the Bureau of Logistics, Department of Health officers in Jakarta told Fritz and Tito that they received no commodities from the GSA orders of February and May. They said they knew when commodities arrived, because USAID gave them copies of the airway bill or ship bill of lading, and they had received none. Fritz later visited USAID, where an Indonesian employee said he had sent several airway bills to the Bureau of Logistics in mid-May. Obviously, communications were not functioning properly. The delivered commodities, scales, a centrifuge, and medicine were picked up by project vehicle in late July and August.

Indonesian government procedures gradually became clearer. When the Bureau of Logistics received an airway bill, it arranged for Customs clearance and placed the commodities in a Department of Health warehouse, after which it notified an officer in the National Institute of Health Research and Development. This officer had the commodities picked up and delivered to his office at the institute. Gradually Tarwotjo and Tito learned the value of paying a call on this gentleman during their weekend visits to Jakarta. However, he had no way of knowing that commodities were in Indonesia until informed by the Bureau of Logistics. The process seemed to require two months.

Fritz again visited USAID on August 15 to see if he could find a way to short-circuit the procedure. He succeeded in obtaining copies of airway bills and warehouse receipts which showed the delivery at Halim of three cartons of surgical instruments and an incubator in late June and their deposit in the Department of Health warehouse on July 23. Fritz and Tito took these documents to the institute, and the responsible officer used them to obtain the equipment from the warehouse. The project supply officer picked them up the following week.

These experiences indicated that the procedure could be accelerated if project officers had access to the relevant documents. Despite repeated verbal requests and an additional letter to USAID on August 23, however, it was never possible to secure these documents from USAID on a routine basis. The responsible Indonesian employee apparently found it difficult to understand the urgency of the matter.

Interim Solutions

What was the project to do in the absence of these commodities? It had to proceed; otherwise it would have been paying salaries and incentives to nearly 100 project employees without any results. Project headquarters began to operate with a typewriter borrowed from the Department of Health and another purchased by HKI. In March 1977, two long carriage typewriters were picked up from USAID. The HKI typewriter was then sold to purchase a refrigerator. Tarwotjo, project manager and head of the Nutrition Academy in Jakarta, borrowed scales from the latter institution until project scales arrived in March. In March the project also purchased with HKI funds a centrifuge and a calculator. It made its old vehicles operational by purchasing tires and batteries and fixing old parts. Between January and September it spent thousands of dollars for the local purchase of medicines and clinical supplies because American requisitions had not yet arrived.

In October 1977 USAID furnished project officers with a status report on the procurement of Demerol ordered in a September 1976 PIO/C. The report stated that Demerol was a controlled substance requiring an import permit. Project officers were advised to obtain a certificate of Official Approval of Import indicating the quantity to be imported, name of importer, authority to import from the United States, and name or designation of the consignee. Since the project had been procuring the drug in Indonesia since Study II began in June and it appeared that the need for the drug would expire before its delivery, project officers advised USAID to cancel the order.

The crucial items, except for the six jeeps, were the USAID supplied slit lamp and the WHO supplied spectrophotometer. By July Study II was in desperate need of a slit lamp, and the project purchased one for Rupiah 1,300,000 ($3,370), paying for it in three installments. In Bogor, Dr. Muhilal performed some ingenious handiwork on his ancient spectrophotometer to make it perform most of the work demanded of it by the project, but no one could predict how long this could continue. Arrival of the new instrument in October was welcomed with open arms. As noted previously, however, it was not operational.

CONTROLS

> Events never develop according to plan; unexpected problems must be met and opportunities seized. (5)

During 1975-1976 a substantial part of AID's Washington manpower was engaged in the development of a new planning, programming, and management information system for the agency. As part of this effort, project managers around the world were asked to plot out in PERT fashion the critical events to occur in their projects. Critical events were defined as those events which had to take place before other desired results could be achieved. If a critical event were one month late, the USAID mission would cable the regional assistant administrator in Washington. If the critical event were postponed by three months, the agency's deputy administrator was to be informed.

If any of the major studies had not been initiated on schedule, it is clear that the government of Indonesia would not have the information it needed for planning nutritional action programs for its third five-year plan (REPELITA III). It is clear also that the project would have no useful information to report to the International Vitamin A Consultative Group meeting scheduled to take place in Brazil in the fall of 1978. The Indonesian Nutritional Blindness Prevention Research Project was beset with problems. These problems were resolved by people working directly on the project, who when necessary sought the assistance of the local USAID mission. These people had enough delegation of authority. They took calculated risks because decisions had to be made whether to proceed or to do nothing. They almost always decided to proceed and to tackle the problems they caused by so doing.

Compliance: Possible Consequences

For a moment, let us suppose that HKI and Indonesian decision makers had decided not to initiate Study II in June 1977 because of the lack of a slit lamp, medicines, and surgical supplies, or let us suppose that they decided they could not start Study IV by October 1 because the jeeps would not arrive in time.

To move the three Study IV teams by October 1, the jeeps would have to arrive in Jakarta no later than September 1 to allow for customs clearance and vehicle registration. This assumes field training of the three teams in August and September with the use of horse wagons, as was done. To assure delivery in Jakarta by September 1, the vehicles should have been shipped from Baltimore by July 15. July 15 was the date of the critical event. On August 15, under the management information system described previously, the USAID mission would have cabled the regional assistant administrator in AID in Washington that the critical event was one month overdue. It is hard to say what action the mission might have recommended to resolve the problem.

Local procurement was already out of the question. In February project officers had already determined that an April order for six jeeps locally assembled could assure delivery of only two in June, two in July, and two in August. Besides, after two months of discussing this issue, the mission had just decided in late March to ask AID in Washington to proceed with original statewide procurement plans, and it is doubtful that the mission would have recommended the expensive proposition of air transportation.

By October 15 the critical event would have become three months old. On September 22 project officers learned that delivery of the jeeps to the port in Baltimore had been further delayed from August 25 to September 20. USAID had known this by late August, but its letter informing the project was postmarked September 8 in Jakarta and was not finally delivered until September 22. Thus, if the agency's deputy administrator had been informed on October 15 that the critical event was three months overdue, it is quite difficult to see what he could have done to remedy the situation. The jeeps were now on the high seas.

If Study IV had not begun when it did, it might never have happened, and the world would have been denied the information it was intended to produce. For one thing, the information was needed by June 1978 for REPELITA III planning, and Indonesian budgets were fixed by this schedule. For another, by August the project had already recruited and put into training the 30 individuals required to conduct the study. It had already taken some months to locate and to entice the senior professionals required. These professionals had been provided by their parent organizations for a limited time period, the time scheduled to conduct the study. Preliminary visits to the 24 provinces had already been made, and the 24 governors had provided clearances for the current schedule. If initiation of Study IV were postponed until arrival of the vehicles, say two months, project officers would have had to reschedule all activities, obtain new clearances, and get consent from the parent organization of the senior professionals to extend their time on the project. If the information could not have been made available for REPELITA III, it is doubtful that the central government would have fully supported rescheduling efforts.

HKI in New York telephoned AID in Washington a number of times on these matters. As it turned out, however, the problems were resolved by communication between project officers and USAID in Jakarta, and Study IV began on time.

PROJECT SCHEDULES

> ...adherence to an implementation schedule is more critical to some types of projects than others. (6)

After this experience in commodity procurement, one may reflect on the lessons learned and how project managers might avoid such hiatuses in the future. As pointed out to the author by Mr. Thomas Niblock, the USAID's Jakarta Mission Director, we have had more than 25 years of experience in aid programs and should have learned by now that United States government procurement is slow and full of pitfalls. Why do we not take this experience into account when we plan technical assistance projects?

While insisting that the U.S. aid program should not be subjected to such intolerable conditions, the author is forced to agree that managers should take realistic cognizance of their existence in project planning and scheduling. But in reviewing the experience of this case study, one is also forced to admit that this was done.

A review of Figure 2.1 will indicate that the planners, HKI and Indonesia, originally anticipated agreement on the project during the early months of 1976. By June 15, when USAID wrote that it was preparing the procurement documents, the government of Indonesia had not yet completed its own clearances for signing the agreement. If this had been done, the USAID procurement documents could have been issued at that time. After the agreement was signed in late August, the Indonesians and HKI personnel geared up to implement the project in the original time frame, forced by the time limits of the HKI contract and the availability of American and Indonesian personnel for specific time periods.

The project is indebted to USAID in Jakarta for the equipment and the extraordinary help in renting Study IV vehicles while awaiting delivery of American jeeps. It is this kind of help which is most appreciated when one encounters the inevitable but unpredictable problems inherent in undertaking international technical assistance activities.

7 Project Funding

BUDGET DEVELOPMENT

Budgeting is an integral part of project development and continuing operations. A logical way to begin in a comprehensive project such as this is to review every step anticipated in the project in considerable detail.

General Preparation

Without reference to possible sources of funding, the budgeter simply lists all resources required for each step during the entire life of the project, whether the nature of such resources is manpower, materials, or services. He then puts a price tag on each item and checks its validity by reference to the market, which includes supplier's catalogues, airline rates, and civil service pay scales. The next step is to determine the sources of funding, preferably on the basis of a previously agreed set of principles regarding the sharing of costs among the recipient country and one or more donor agencies. What has now become two or more budgets must each be divided into annual budgets which coincide with the fiscal years of each participating agency. At this stage, one must be able to predict whether the amounts needed will be available within the appropriation process of each agency. Subsequently, these annual budgets are further divided into quarterly and monthly operating budgets, at which time realism is tested in the actual available flow of funds.

A longstanding principle in technical assistance budgeting is that the donor pays for external costs (those goods and services to be imported) while the host government pays local costs. At different times and places, the principle has been rigidly enforced by external donors. To a large extent, the principle has been relaxed to reflect the realities which exist in certain countries and for certain projects. In other countries, where the governments can afford it, they are asked to pay for some or all of the external requirements of a technical assistance project.

Indonesian Budget

In August 1975, Tarwotjo, Sommer, and Dr. Susan Pettiss prepared the first gross budget which is summarized in Table 7.1. This table reflects a renumbering of the studies included in the 1975 gross budget so that they coincide with the usage finally developed. The original budget did not include a study comparable to what is now Study III.

This project in Indonesia, if to be successful, required considerable relaxation of the technical assistance budgeting principle. Though Indonesia seemed inherently rich in resources, these had never been fully developed. Though long a colony, even now only a small fraction of rural children were able to go to school for more than several years. Many years of hyperinflation and bad economic management during the 1950s and early 1960s had wasted resources and destroyed economic initiative. The present government was making a determined effort to bring about stability and restore the nation's credit in the international marketplace. The rise in oil prices had relieved the situation somewhat, because Indonesia was blessed with this resource. However, this blessing had to be spread over a very large, growing population. The task of creating and spreading educational and employment opportunities and health benefits was gigantic, and budgets continued to be extremely tight. The dimensions of the problems are signified by the growing proportion of youngsters in the population. By 1980 65% will be under 25 years of age.

Other considerations related to cost-sharing were the special measures discussed in Chapter 3 for attracting able Indonesians to the project. For the most part they left permanent parent organizations to accept temporary leadership positions with the project. Some left lucrative private medical practices performed in addition to government jobs. In some cases they continued to perform their permanent functions on a part-time basis. The sacrifices demanded by the project required incentives in addition to the continuation of low government salaries.

Table 7.1. Summary of First Project Budget, August 1975

STUDY I	$ 509,025
Personnel (25 persons for 15-28 months, 1-26 months, 3-25 months, 4-4 months, 2 local aides).	275,250
Equipment and supplies (2 jeeps, insurance, gas and oil, scales, printing forms, centrifuge, incubator freezer, furniture, miscellaneous).	67,775
Other expenses (punch cards, computer, serum vitamin A, bacterial cultures, incentives, printing and publishing, reprints, hospitalization of cases, internal meetings).	166,000
STUDY II	$ 170,573
Personnel (7 persons for 24 months).	108,900
Equipment and supplies (1 jeep, insurance, gas and oil, scales, printing forms, miscellaneous).	25,223
Other expenses (punch cards, computer, serum vitamin A, bacterial cultures, hospitalization, printing and publishing, travel).	36,450
STUDY IV	$ 327,410
Personnel (three teams: 12 persons each for 8 months).	199,200
Equipment and supplies (rental of jeeps and motorcycles, gas and oil, forms, scales, miscellaneous).	50,970
Other expenses (punch cards, computer, public transport, supervisory trips, printing and publishing, reprints, international meetings).	77,240
SPECIAL STUDIES	$ 83,876
GENERAL SUPPORT	$ 387,383
Personnel (19 persons including 1 foreigner, for 36 months, not including the steering committee).	286,000
Equipment and supplies (2 jeeps, VW bus, insurance, gas and oil, office equipment, 6 typewriters, 2 calculators, miscellaneous).	84,100
Other expenses (postage, telegraph, telephone, xerox rental, international travel).	17,383
TOTAL	$1,487,267

Finally, the project was of international significance. Research results obtained in Indonesia would be available to other developing countries which experienced eye disease caused by vitamin A deficiency. Thus, donor agencies had a strong interest in achieving promised research results. The Indonesian government, while keenly interested in the project, could not have undertaken the whole package without extraordinary relaxation in the principles of cost sharing.

Despite such relaxation, Indonesian project planners in August 1975 were despondent about chances of obtaining the Indonesian government funds required. Estimates over the life of the project ranged upward from $500, 000. Such sums appeared impossible to obtain because ceilings for government expenditures had been frozen for the remainder of the current five-year plan. During this agonizing reappraisal, planners recalled a prior decision to postpone expanded mass distribution of vitamin A capsules until they had the research results. By referring to plans for expanded distribution, they located the funds necessary to carry out the research.

Budget Revisions

Over the next months both Indonesian government planners and HKI planners in the United States attempted to refine the original gross budget, splitting the costs between HKI and the Indonesian government and phasing expenditures over several fiscal years. Of course the fiscal years were different; the Indonesian government's year ran from May through April and the HKI year from July through June. These budgets are summarized in Table 7.2.

In September 1975, less than a month after the departure of HKI planners, Tarwotjo informed New York that he had already submitted the proposal to his ministry. HKI copies of his comprehensive budget tables delineated both Indonesian government and external costs by fiscal year and included basic data on Indonesian government salaries, per diem, local, and external incentive scales, as well as information on travel, use of supplies, etc. He projected total costs at $1,451,959, very close to the previous jointly formulated budget, allocating $360,973 to the Indonesian government and $1,090,986 to external costs. While Tarwotjo's schedule assumed project approval in January 1976, he projected real project activity to begin in September of that year.

Another HKI budget found in project files is undated, but was based on Tarwotjo's budget described previously. It projects some Indonesian staff on the job in January 1976, with major Study I work to begin in April and to continue into fiscal year (FY) 1979. Total project costs amounted to $2,089,475, split between $1,586,892 for

Table 7.2. Comparison of Early Project Budgets
($1,000)

	Consultant August 1975	Indonesian Government September 1975	HKI September 1975	Indonesian Government January 1976	HKI February 1976	Indonesian Government May 1976
Indonesian Government		361	503	551	551	423
External		1,091	1,056	646	649	644
HKI Technical Assistance			530		588	
TOTAL	1,478	1,452	2,089	1,197	1,788	1,067

external donors and $502,583 for the Indonesian government. This included an item for HKI technical assistance and support amounting to $530,975, an item not included in Indonesian government budgets.

In January 1976, Tarwotjo sent a revised budget to HKI in NY. His budget again reflected a more realistic judgment of the project's launching date, projecting expenditures to begin in September 1976 and to end in June 1979. Projections of total costs were lower than previous budgets, with larger Indonesian government costs and much smaller estimates of external costs.

Anxious to present a reasonably firm budget to AID for contractual purposes, HKI's new budget of February 2, 1976 accepted Tarwotjo's latest figures, only adding amounts required for HKI technical assistance. Dates were more realistic, showing no real project activity until September 1976.

HKI officers visited Indonesia twice during early 1976 to firm up budget and other project plans. Part of their anxiety was caused by the Indonesian government's recognition of the overextended operations and international obligations to the government's petroleum organization, Pertamina. Earlier, when it seemed that rising oil prices could contribute mightily to development efforts, ministries had been encouraged to increase their budgets. Under the latest BAPPENAS (Indonesian planning agency) reviews, however, new project proposals were eliminated and the budgets of many continuing projects were slashed. HKI officers were naturally concerned that this new project might be eliminated. Health Department officials were successful, however, in their insistence that the project was a continuing activity, a natural follow-up to previous collaboration with HKI, and the budget remained relatively unscathed. Perhaps, however, these reviews caused health officers to hold their estimates to the minimum.

Tarwotjo continued to review and reconstruct the budget with government budget officers. After review with the director of the National Health Research and Development Institute, he forwarded the latest revised budget to HKI in May. This budget showed still lower total costs, this time by decreasing Indonesian government costs. Conveniently for HKI, he showed comparisons between this budget and his January version and explained the revisions.

For Study I, a new regulation decreased Indonesian costs by lowering per diem rates. External costs were raised by an item not previously included, compensation for "loss of medical practice."

Revisions in the Study II budget contained a supervisory nurse and pediatrician not previously included, thus raising both Indonesian and external costs. Study III contained higher Indonesian and lower external costs. Indonesian government planners had added per diem costs for extra field supervisors, but had eliminated other costs in fiscal year 1979, presumably on the assumption that computer analysis would be completed prior to that time.

The Study IV budget revised the schedule as well as financing, reflecting the Indonesian desire to use results of the national prevalence survey in developing the third Five Year Plan (REPELITA III). Preliminary travel and purchase of equipment were shoved forward from FY 1977-78 to FY 1976-77. The bulk of activity was programmed for FY 1977-78, causing increases that year of $10,000 and $38,000 for Indonesian and external costs, respectively. Incentive rates for nurse-enumerators were raised significantly. Unfortunately, however, the budgeters had reduced travel costs drastically, assuming that nurse-enumerators could be recruited locally in each province. This assumption ignored the timing required for recruiting and training such nurse-enumerators and the problems of correcting errors for many different people in different locations. On the basis of this unworkable assumption, the overall Study IV budget had been reduced $31,000 and $20,000 for Indonesian government and external costs, respectively. However, Tarwotjo indicated in his letter that the proposal was unworkable, thus leaving open the possibility that it would be corrected. Tarwotjo also pointed out an error in the revised general support budget, which reduced Indonesian costs by $81,000. Budgeters had omitted costs of the steering committee in the revised budget. As it turned out, the head of the National Health Research Institute had approved this deletion in order to provide for higher salaries of staff and meeting expenses.

It will be recalled from Chapter 2 that the initial HKI-AID contract was signed May 28, 1977. Just 14 days prior to this, HKI in NY received Tarwotjo's revised budget which contained errors already recognized by the Indonesians. Given the long distance communications involved and the considerable doubts about the Indonesian government's budgetary intentions, as well as HKI budgetary requirements, one wonders at HKI boldness in proceeding without additional joint planning sessions in Indonesia.

Involvement with Other Agencies

> Organizations may reduce possible environmental controls and maximize their autonomy by forming exchange relationships with many and diverse units of their task environment that can provide needed resources. (1)

To complicate matters, HKI desired to hold down its contract costs by engaging other participants, such as WHO, UNICEF, and USAID in Jakarta, in the effort. Thus most external commodity requirements became the responsibility of those agencies. On the face of it, this would relieve HKI personnel of much responsibility. A contrary conclusion may be drawn from Chapter 6. However, it is possible that the principle quoted above may still have operated to the project's advantage.

As revised on September 30, 1976, the contract AID in Washington provided a total budget support of HKI project operations of $1,093,185 as indicated in Table 7.3.

Until June 30, 1976, the United States government's fiscal year was on a July-June basis. Beginning with October 1976, the United States government's fiscal year changed to an October-September system. However, since the bulk of contract funds were obligated by AID in FY 1976 and the interim quarter, HKI did not have to consider this difference in further budget negotiations.

BUDGETARY PROBLEMS

> The nature of development is such that what is predictable is unpredictability. (2)

HKI had anticipated spending considerable funds of its own in addition to those supplied by AID. It naturally wanted to minimize such expenditures because it had to finance these mainly from private contributions.

After Dr. Sommer arrived in Indonesia in late August 1976, he, Tarwotjo, and Tito reviewed all budgetary sources item by item. After considering all possible economic measures, they calculated a remaining shortfall of approximately $100-125,000. There were basically three causes for this situation:

1. Indonesian government budgeters had omitted some large items such as $30,000 needed for air tickets for preliminary planning visits for Study IV to the provinces. The Indonesian Planning Agency (BAPPENAS) had approved the final budgetary figures, so apparently total Indonesian expenditures as well as annual expenditures were fixed. Moreover, there were limitations to maneuvering within these fixed boundaries. HKI officers had pointed out to Tarwotjo this omission in his May budget, but were reluctant to be too demanding lest this result in delaying or scuttling the government agreement. (3)

2. Prior calculations of per diem costs were based on up to 30 days per diem per month. It turned out to be an Indonesian government rule, however, to pay a maximum of 18 days per diem per month, to be used for payment of transportation as well as food and lodging.

Table 7.3. AID-HKI Contract Budget, September 30, 1976

Category	June 1, 1976-December 31, 1976	January 1, 1977-December 31, 1977	January 1, 1978-December 31, 1978	January 1, 1979-July 31, 1979	Total
American salaries and wages	$ 45,220	$ 72,800	$ 73,550	$ 37,100	$ 228,670
Local salaries and wages	42,097	117,980	123,635	28,045	311,575
Allowances	24,608	34,220	34,220	14,465	107,513
Materials and equipment	6,950	14,450	15,250	2,500	39,150
International travel per diem and storage	16,250	8,250	20,250	20,800	65,550
Local travel including gas, oil, and maintenance	6,500	31,870	36,000	5,500	79,870
Other direct costs	2,950	21,530	84,630	25,800	134,910
Subtotal	144,575	301,100	387,535	134,210	967,420
Overhead	18,795	39,143	50,380	17,447	125,765
Total	$ 163,370	$ 340,243	$ 437,915	$ 151,657	$1,093,185

3. Estimates used in contract negotiations for gasoline and vehicle maintenance were unrealistically low in view of rising costs. In view of inflationary trends in Indonesia, the consultant had originally recommended a 20% annual contingency factor. Why was this eliminated in contract negotiations? Did AID refuse to consider it, or was HKI reluctant to submit it for fear that AID would turn it down?

At this stage, October 1976, HKI was unwilling to renegotiate its AID contract, just amended on September 30. (4)

Other budgetary worries ensued. A typing error had resulted in deleting the Indonesian government's budgetary provision for telephones. During the life of the project it depended on a single telephone tied to the hospital switchboard. Frequently, the wrong number was called, resulting in hospital and project personnel traipsing across the hospital to take calls and relay messages. This kind of situation is hard to envision by AID officers in Washington, where there is a telephone on each desk. Moreover, the telephone don't always work in Bandung.

The long supply pipeline also raised the vehicle maintenance and other budgetary concerns discussed in Chapter 6. Since phasing of human and material resources is usually better coordinated by a single responsible agent, these concerns might have been avoided by a contractual provision for HKI purchase of the commodities subsequently financed by USAID in Jakarta and purchased by the U. S. General Services Administration (GSA). The use of USAID's Jakarta funds contained a built-in delaying factor, because they were derived from funds allocated to health research in Indonesia. The many competing demands for these funds forced a review and decision each time USAID proposed that a portion be spent for project purposes. This was not the largest delaying factor, however; the primary factor was the extraordinary lapse in time between USAID financing and actual GSA purchase. The secondary factor was the delay within Indonesia after delivery.

There were also some Indonesian government technicalities to be overcome. Budgetary presentations were made for a project entitled "Characterization of Vitamin A Deficiency and Xerophthalmia in Indonesia." When the project got underway, it seemed more practical to entitle it simply the "Nutritional Blindness Prevention Project." When interview and examination forms were printed with use of the latter title, Indonesian finance officers refused to pay. How this problem was solved is a secret of the project. More serious was the price of the forms which apparently was raised by the 33-1/3% contribution expected of the printing firm.

The sources of procurement was another technicality. During project development, Bandung prices had been used to calculate costs of office furniture and equipment, but after the project started, the market for private purchases proved an unsuitable indicator for costs of official purchases. The Jakarta money controllers insisted that office equipment be purchased in Jakarta, where prices were not only 25% higher but involved additional costs for transportation to Bandung. This policy was resisted but not overcome. Of course, these technicalities only applied to Indonesian government expenditures, not to those of HKI.

The project had difficulty in covering the costs of Study IV travel to the provinces. The Indonesian budget presentation for FY 1977-78 spoke of six zones rather than 24 provinces; thus, finance people in Jakarta had to be convinced that approval really covered the latter.

PROCEDURES

Funds filtered to the project in several ways. USAID in Jakarta, WHO, and UNICEF funds for equipment purchases were for the project, of course, but were never handled by the project's finance officer. Salaries of Indonesian professional employees who also worked for parent institutions were paid directly by those institutions. Salaries of HKI American employees were paid directly into American bank accounts. The Department of Health in Jakarta paid some expenses directly, where evidence was furnished for the service performed. For this purpose, the project submitted to the department one copy of every telegram sent as evidence of its expenditure. When paying per diem, gasoline, and other expenses, Tito picked up funds from the department periodically during weekend visits to Jakarta.

HKI in New York transferred funds to the project by an indirect route. Each month HKI authorized Citibank in New York to transfer funds to an HKI dollar account in Jakarta in amounts designed to meet requirements forecast in quarterly projections prepared in Bandung. They also purchased some equipment and supplies directly and mailed or shipped them to the project, and they disbursed funds in New York for home office support and overhead.

About the middle of each month HKI officers in Bandung transferred funds from Citibank in Jakarta to the project account in Bank Bumi Daya in Bandung which were sufficient to cover payments due through the early part of the following month. Incentives and compensation for loss of medical practice were generally paid on the first of the month by the project finance officer, an Indonesian who also managed the project account. Unlike most modern endeavors in the United States, most project payments were in cash. Few people in

Indonesia know what to do with a check. In fact, most people would be suspect if checks were found in their possession.

A review of one monthly payroll operation exemplifies some anomalies. Fritz invited the Price Waterhouse affiliate in Jakarta to send an auditor to Bandung on Monday, October 3, 1977, to observe the payroll operation. Over the long distance telephone, this representative asked Fritz how many project employees would be paid. Fritz expected 49 persons to appear for payment, but mentioned the impossibility of paying all employees in one place on one day. Many employees would not be present.

In an early morning conversation with Fritz and Soemantri, the finance officer, the auditor opined that this operation was somewhat unusual; he was accustomed to observing factory payroll operations where it was easier to account for persons who did not show up. Soemantri wrote a check for several million rupiah countersigned by Dr. Sugana, project clinical investigator and director of Cicendo. Soemantri went to the bank, drew out the cash, returned to the office and counted out the money in individual piles which he put into envelopes.

Members of the Study I team lined up first. Facing a two or three hour drive before they could begin the day's field work, they were in a rush. Each employee signed his name on three copies of the appropriate payroll sheet and was given his money. After the Study I team finished, the Study II team and general support staff appeared for their pay. At the end of the process, the auditor asked project officers to account for the 38 missing persons.

Asikin Yusuf.

The first was Dr. Zein Sulaiman, who had recently replaced Dr. Yusuf as pediatrician on the Study I team. And this seems as good a place as any to relate the Dr. Yusuf saga.

Dr. Yusuf's release to the project had been negotiated with the local medical faculty and hospital director sometime before the beginning of the Study I base line clinical round. He joined the Study I team in March 1977, moving into a room of the project's subheadquarters in Purwakarta. From the anticipated per diem, he paid a large share of the two-year cost of renting this building, because leases are commonly paid in advance in Indonesia. Unfortunately, project officers did not realize that the hospital had no right to assign Dr. Yusuf to the project. Hardly had he moved in and begun work before his parent organization, the Directorate General of Medical Services, ordered him to report to Jakarta for reassignment.

Dr. Yusuf, an experienced field worker, looked forward to completing two years on the project. Unmarried, he spent his weekends at his home in Bandung. Project officials disliked changing personnel in the midst of a research project, but their request for rescinding the order was denied. The matter was taken to the project head, Professor Sulianti Sarosa, whose request also was denied. She suggested that Dr. Yusuf not move as yet, however, as the Directorate General of Medical Services must name a replacement for her clearance, and her standards would be high. By August, however, it became clear that Yusuf would have to leave the project. The directorate general named Dr. Zein, who had excellent qualifications, to replace him. Dr. Zein appeared on the scene and rented a house for his family in Purwakarta. Since he would use his per diem to rent his family house, the project reimbursed Dr. Yusuf for his advance payments from HKI funds, feeling that Dr. Yusuf should not have to bear this as a personal loss. This amount, of course, had not been budgeted.

Dr. Zein understudied Dr. Yusuf during part of September, and the project petitioned a delay in Yusuf's reassignment until the end of October so that Yusuf could replace Dr. Tien Tamba, Study II pediatrician, during the latter's upcoming maternity leave. He managed to understudy Dr. Tien for several days before she was forced to go to the general hospital for her delivery. Thus, HKI funded an extra position during September and October. In November, when Dr. Yusuf reported to Jakarta for reassignment, he was informed that the directorate general had rescinded its order on the basis of Professor Sulianti's objections. Having nowhere else to go, Dr. Yusuf returned to his job at the Bandung Hospital. Several months later he was transferred to Karawang, but he continued his interest in the project.

Additional staffing - budgetary difficulties.

On October 3, Dr. Zein did not make the trip from Purwakarta to get paid. He wrote a note to Dr. Hussaini saying that his wife was ill; however, he would be available for field work after the team returned from Bandung.

Dr. Tien Tamba, happy with her baby, did not appear for payment as was true of two other employees who were ill. Then there were the Study IV teams, all 27 members, who had departed for Bali on September 30. All of them had been paid on the 29th, as had Tarwotjo, Tito, and Djoko, the project supervisors who accompanied the three teams during their initial week of operations. From then on, payment in Bandung for Study IV personnel would be a rare occasion. After completing the islands of Bali and Lombok, they struck across Java in three separate paths going from east to west, after which they headed for separate Outer Islands.

Professor Sulianti Sarosa, head of the project, was officed in Jakarta and often was out of the country. The finance officer never met her. Her name was on a separate payroll sheet which Tarwotjo took to Jakarta once a month. If he secured her signature, he paid her.

Then there were the three doctors who headed the hospital in Purwakarta and two community health centers in the Study I area of operations. They kept special records on xerophthalmia patients, dispensed vitamin A pills, and referred corneal cases to the Study II Clinic. The first received Rupiah 10,000 ($25) and the latter two doctors received Rupiah 5,000 each per month.

On October 5, Soemantri went to Purwakarta and paid Dr. Zein. Learning of a meeting that day which the three other doctors expected to attend, he headed for that meeting and paid two of the doctors. The third, not in attendance, was also not present at the community health center when Soemantri visited. He returned to Bandung about 8 P.M. feeling that he had not completed his job.

In Bogor, a three-hour drive from Bandung, Dr. Muhilal collected Rupiah 50,000 ($125) monthly to share among five lab technicians who worked overtime for the project. It appeared unreasonable for the lab technicians to endure a six-hour round trip to Bandung each month, or for the finance officer to go to Bogor once a month. It seemed far more practical for Djoko, the project statistician, to carry the funds with him during his Friday night return to Bogor at the same time he delivered frozen blood to his next door neighbor, Muhilal. It also seemed more practical for Tito, Djoko, or Tarwotjo to convey funds to the three doctors in the Purwakarta area during their supervisory and consulting visits to that area. Though perhaps not good payroll procedures, practical approaches were needed.

A longer range procedure was worked out for paying the Study IV teams which were continually moving from one sample site to another. Project officers arranged to transfer funds to bank accounts in the names of the three team leaders, along with vehicle registration numbers, in the regency city nearest to project operations on payday. The team leaders paid team members and mailed the signed payroll sheets to Bandung.

Initial Budgetary Outlays

A small voluntary agency like HKI, dependent on private contributions, assumes a substantial financial risk when it takes on a comprehensive venture like Vitamin A Blindness Prevention Research in Indonesia. True, it was reimbursed by AID for the larger portion of its outlay.

However, it had to make the outlay first through the Citibank account, for example, then await expenditure reports from Indonesia before billing AID. It then awaited reimbursement. The intervening period could last several months.

Some of the HKI outlays were quite substantial. For example, per Indonesia custom it advanced rent on houses for the two HKI American employees for the duration of the project, but it was unable to bill AID for these advance expenditures, and billed AID as if the outlay was on a monthly rental basis. HKI also advanced funds for the purchase of automobiles for the official use of these employees and did not claim reimbursement for these expenditures. The outlays were a substantial amount for HKI to carry over such a long period.

These HKI advance outlays were exacerbated somewhat by the advent of Study IV. The Indonesian government was responsible for all per diem payments. However, the project was unable to secure Indonesian funds for this purpose until the third or fourth of the month, sometimes later. Two separate bank transfer operations for the Study IV teams each month would involve six different banks, double the transfer costs, and require each of the three team leaders to take time out from fast moving project operations on two separate days to visit a bank, verify his credentials, collect the funds, and pay his team members. It was far simpler and more efficient for HKI to advance project funds for per diem, amalgamating this advance with other salaries and incentives for one payroll transfer transaction. The project account was then reimbursed after receipt of Indonesian per diem funds. The additional outlay each month for this purpose amounted to nearly $5,000.

Transportation Equipment

An item of considerable concern, once it became clear that the six USAID-financed jeeps would not arrive in time to begin Study IV, was whether HKI would be forced to expend its own funds for the local rental of vehicles. On August 9, 1977, Dr. A. Sommer, project scientist, wrote to the director of USAID in Jakarta pointing out the circumstances caused by the earlier three-month hold order USAID had imposed on vehicle procurement. The project had been frozen into its present schedule. All professional and field workers had been recruited and were in training. The professionals were limited in the time they were available. Clearances had been received from 24 provincial governors for the scheduled visits. Moreover, any delay would result in unavailability of the survey data and recommendations for inclusion in the government's third five-year plan. He asked for USAID assistance.

At the request of the responsible USAID officer, Fritz visited USAID on September 8. USAID had located $17,101 which it could agree to spend on transportation for the project. In a long-distance telephone conversation on Friday, September 23, the same officer said that a letter of agreement was being prepared, and would be sent for Indonesian government signature to the National Institute for Health Research and Development either that day or on Monday, September 26.

Meanwhile, project officers had been negotiating a contract with a Bandung transportation firm. Arrangements were made to sign the contract on September 28, so the Study IV teams could begin their move to Bali on September 30. The contractor agreed to a delay in initial payment, but insisted on receiving a copy of the signed letter of agreement as a guarantee. On September 26, Fritz went to the National Institute in Jakarta to make sure the agreement was signed and to get a copy. Unfortunately, the agreement had not yet been received. Fritz telephoned USAID and asked about the agreement. While the USAID officer was "checking," the long-distance operator interrupted the call and Fritz was unable to get another call through to USAID, so he drove there.

Arriving at USAID, Fritz was told that the letter was "in USAID clearance." Fritz checked with all responsible USAID officers who had not yet seen it. Discussing the matter with a secretary, he discovered the letter had not yet been typed. After it was typed, he personally took the letter through the USAID clearance gauntlet and secured an official letter number from the USAID communications section. Since National Institute offices were closed for the day, Fritz took the letter to Tarwotjo's house and asked him to convey it to Professor Sulianti for signature the next morning. The next morning Professor Sulianti Sarosa was in a meeting with the Minister of Health, and it had every appearance of lasting all day. However, when Fritz and Tarwotjo returned to the National Institute that afternoon, an officer produced a copy of the signed agreement. He had boldly invaded the minister's meeting, and obtained Professor Sulianti's signature.

The contractor received his guarantee, but this was not the end of the matter. There was still a wait before USAID funds were received. Upon receipt of the signed agreement from Professor Sulianti, USAID was expected to issue a check. The institute would transfer these funds to the project bank account, account for all funds expended, and return funds unused by the time the six jeeps were delivered.

On October 6, Tarwotjo called Fritz from Jakarta, reporting that a visit to USAID had revealed that the check had to be issued in Bangkok. On a later visit by Fritz on October 14, he was told the check was due but had not yet been received. The next day Tito arranged to borrow limited funds from another account of the National Institute, but was told this exceptional practice could not be repeated. After another call to Jakarta on October 24 revealed that the check still had not been received, Fritz consented to a temporary withdrawal of HKI project funds to pay for Study IV's transportation, which would be reimbursed by USAID funds through the National Institute.

These events make it clear that USAID officers wanted to be helpful. They came through with the necessary funds. It is equally clear, however, that only project personnel really perceived the emergency they were in and were sufficiently free from organizational and procedural rigidities to take the actions required. The donor organization, organized for worldwide "efficient" conduct of United States operations, is not geared to the solving of single project emergencies. The following is quoted from a USAID letter received during the midst of these difficulties:

> I am glad we in USAID have been able to help you follow your plans as closely as possible and regret the problems generated from delays in vehicle procurement. I'm sure, however, that you have become aware that such delays are almost to be expected, and that slippages of a few weeks in work schedules are not unique.

AID Reviews

Sometimes AID in Washington reviews of project expenditures caused delays in reimbursement. For the first year, HKI in New York submitted its claims directly to the AID contracting officer. In June 1977, a new regulation required prior clearance from the Office of Nutrition project officer, and problems ensued. In September 1977, the HKI director of blindness prevention wrote that AID was still questioning costs related to the shipment of household effects the previous January, but had agreed to release three months of reimbursement, approximately $109,000, on the understanding that these questions would be resolved the following month. In November she wrote that HKI's reimbursement claim had been lost in AID for the second time and that HKI was taking steps to establish a credit line for future borrowing in advance of reimbursements.

These financial pressures were a continuous stimulant to HKI in New York to hold to a minimum its transfers to Citibank in Jakarta. Project officers in Bandung felt, on the other hand, that the account should consistently be high enough to cover contingencies, including the contingency that a transfer from New York would be delayed. Neither party was ever fully satisfied with the balance achieved.

Indonesian Government Procedures

Another interesting feature of project funding was the trade-off aspect. Occasionally, Indonesian personnel found their government's budgetary restrictions too confining. Sometimes it appeared that some project operations would have to be closed down unless HKI came to the rescue. One example was the interview and examination forms. The government budgeted for these and for card-punching; HKI was to pay for computer programming. Early in fiscal 1977-78, however, the expenses for forms exceeded the government's budget. On the other hand, Indonesian project officers found they were allowed to use some of their government card punching funds for computer programming. Thus, a trade-off was accomplished.

A similar problem was encountered for the agreed division of costs between gasoline and vehicle maintenance. In this case the government ruled that a proportion of its vehicle expenses must be for maintenance. So, it was agreed informally that HKI and the government would split costs of both gasoline and maintenance. The 1977-78 budget for the telephone, however, only amounted to Rupiah 50,000 ($125) for the entire year. The director of the Cicendo Hospital, also clinical investigator of the project, agreed to carry the costs of the telephone if the project defrayed Study II hospitalization costs. A typical hospitalization thus involved (a) conveyance by public vehicle of the patient from a rural community health center to the Study I team in Purwakarta which was reimbursed from HKI funds, (b) conveyance by Study I jeep to Cicendo with gasoline paid by either the government or HKI, (c) hospitalization paid by the government's project budget, and (d) return of the patient and parent to home by project vehicle with gasoline paid to the extent permitted from the government's budget, otherwise by HKI.

Government officials were appreciative of this flexibility on the part of HKI. It is interesting to conjecture what would have happened if the HKI hirelings, not really representatives of the agency but merely contracted employees, had referred these trade-offs to New York for a decision. Quite possibly, the project would have had to fold, at least temporarily, on a number of occasions.

A school of thought in technical assistance sets forth the principle that the donor should never take action which relieves the recipient of the necessity to solve his own problems. In general, the author is sympathetic with this view. Indonesian activities are entangled in much red tape. In the long run it will be advantageous to Indonesian development and the Indonesian people if this red tape can be disentangled. Any time a donor agency takes action which overcomes an immediate obstacle caused by built-in government restrictions, the day of government action to remove those restrictions is further postponed.

On the other hand, agencies which pursue this school of thought must learn to bear the consequences. Can a project afford to wait while the machinery of government deliberates complex reform measures, and what incentives does it offer to get the ball rolling? Can the targets of the project be achieved subsequently? Can the agency's contract and agreement be renewed? What happens to project relationships and to the morale of both local and foreign personnel while project activity remains in the doldrums? The principled technical assistance practitioner sometimes faces dilemmas.

In this case study, the primary interest of the technical assistance agency, HKI, was the project at hand. Overall Indonesian administrative problems would have to be solved by agencies more suited to the task. At the time this manuscript was finally typed, HKI expenditures on the project were still in line with its contract with AID. There was no cost overrun.

8 Study IV: The Nationwide Prevalence Survey

PREPARATIONS

> In any country or area, a sizeable intervention program is called for only when Vitamin A deficiency is known to be widespread. (1)

Study IV presented logistical problems of the first order. Its aims were far-reaching: to conduct a countrywide survey of the prevalence of anterior segment ocular pathology, and particularly vitamin A-related corneal disease, among children up to six years of age in the islands of Java, Sumatra, Sulawesi, Kalimantan, Lombok, Bali, and Ambon and to ascertain its relationship to agricultural and dietary patterns and to socioeconomic status of the respective regional populations. Three teams were to conduct the survey, visiting altogether 324 sample sites to examine a nationwide total of 45,000 preschool children.

The original proposal divided the country into six zones. Each zone contained 54 sample sites and a total of 7,500 children to be examined, as indicated in Table 8.1.

The choice of 7,500 children per zone was intended to satisfy the competing priorities between statistical requirements and the practical constraints of time, money, and personnel. In order to obtain useful data for planning purposes, it was necessary to select sample sites by a stratified multistage technique with a probability proportionate to size. To select an appropriate sampling frame, project planners during the early months of 1977 studied the manual used by the Inter Censal Survey and discussed its methodology with officers of the Central Bureau of Statistics in Jakarta. Project officers

Table 8.1. Selecting Study IV Sample Sites

Area	Number of Sample Sites	Number of Children
Java: East	54	7500
Central	54	7500
West	54	7500
Sumatra	54	7500
Sulawesi	54	7500
Kalimantan	24	3750
Lombok	10	1250
Bali	12	1250
Ambon	8	1250
	324	45,000

---

satisfied themselves that these sampling methods met Study IV requirements. A scientific sampling of that survey's sample sites could be used as areas of operation for the Study IV teams.

There was a problem, however; another project was anxious to use the same system for selection of sample sites. If the other project made its selection first, selection of Study IV sites would be restricted to other, probably unrepresentative sample sites. If this turned out to be the case, project officers would have to spend the next two months constructing their sample sites from scratch. To avoid this possibility, project officers succeeded in borrowing the only copy of the bureau's master list for a week to have it xeroxed. They then spent three long days in Bandung constructing the list of Study IV sites. On the basis of field experience to date and a more careful examination of the routes to be followed, they reduced the sites in the five major zones to 40 and increased the number in Lombok, by then recognized as a famine area. They presented the list to the Central Statistics Bureau in Jakarta the following Saturday, thus preempting it from the competing project. Further negotiations with the bureau led to the procurement of necessary site identification data and maps. As it turned out, this flurry of activity was unnecessary. Four months later project officers learned that the competing project had not yet selected its sample.

During April, official letters sent to all provinces explained the aims of the study and the inclusion of the particular province, tentatively scheduled a short preliminary visit by project officers during June-July, and requested that a local Health Department counterpart be available with maps so that travel routes and schedules could be worked out at that time. Favorable replies were received from all governors. At this point, however, travel funds were not yet available because of technicalities associated with an earlier error of budget presentation. After project personnel attended a couple of meetings in Jakarta, funds finally became available.

While awaiting funds, project planners used the intervening period to good advantage in preparing forms and instructions for their use. For previous studies, forms and instructions had been written first in English, then translated and printed in Indonesian. For Study IV Tarwotjo designed the forms and instructions on his own, briefly pausing to review his work with the American project scientist in mid-June. By the end of June, final drafts were nearly ready, and in early July Tarwotjo was seen with a small tape recorder testing some of his nutritional questions at a Study II field site. In late July all Study IV forms and instructions were finally printed in Indonesian before Fritz translated them into English.

Prior to late June it appeared that two ophthalmologists were assured; only one more was needed. At that point, however, a strong protest by one of the parent institutions resulted in the loss of one of the supposedly assured ophthalmologists, so Dr. Sugana had to make a rush recruitment trip across Java during July. Fortunately, he succeeded in obtaining the two additional ophthalmologists required.

By mid-July funds became available for the preliminary visits to the provinces. Time was now too short for all trips to be made by project personnel, so three officers from the Health Department were mobilized to assist in the effort. After a short letter confirming the dates of the visits, six officers proceeded to 24 provinces during late July and early August. Their instructions were to leave nothing to chance. Everything must be ready to move when the survey teams showed up at a later date. Since transportation and communications were obvious problems, these were emphasized. Project managers didn't want to undertake impossible tasks, so they discussed whether or not it was practical to store blood for later shipment.

General Instructions

Their instructions were to leave nothing to chance. Having learned well the lessons of Study I, instructions emphasized the importance of touching base with all people whose support and participation were required. Finally, the following instructions, originally prepared the previous April, were highly specific, aimed at leaving no doubts in the minds of those who were to carry them out:

I. Obtain official permission for survey.

1. Meet the local counterpart.

2. Visit the governor's office.

3. Visit the province's representative from the Health Department.

4. Determine exactly what permission is needed, from whom, and when it must be gotten. All permissions must be ready before the team arrives. The team must be able to begin work <u>immediately</u>. The counterpart is responsible for arranging all permissions not formally obtained during site visit.

II. Arrange for facilities and logistics.

1. At minimum, maps must be available which indicate roads and all sample villages, so work routes and timing can be discussed with the counterpart. Village maps showing the cluster sites should also be obtained. If not yet available, arrange to have the counterpart send them to project headquarters <u>as soon as possible</u>.

2. Using these maps, the counterpart should advise of best work routes in order to cover all sites in the least amount of time (roads to take, starting-off place, order of visits). Try not to double back, unless that's the fastest or only route.

3. Determine estimated travel time to each site from preceding site or overnight stopping point. This includes travel by boat or foot to the actual cluster. Any site that will take <u>more</u> than one day to reach <u>and more</u> than one day to move to next site should be dropped, i.e., if travel time to and from a site is three or more days, not counting work time at the site.

4. Set up an approximate schedule, and determine the most appropriate places for the team to spend the night (in the village itself so they can be warned ahead of time, a nearby town, etc).

5. Discuss the needs at each site: local regency counterpart, a local aide per cluster. The counterpart should make these arrangements.

6. Determine the feasibility of adequately storing blood specimens, i.e., do the sites or overnight stops have electricity, refrigeration, and facilities for getting ice?

7. What is shortest time to ship blood samples from the field to Jakarta at weekly intervals?

8. What is the best means of shipping forms at weekly or biweekly intervals to Jakarta: messenger, the express parcel service, etc.?

9. What is the surest means of communicating from the field to Bandung from each place along the way at least on weekly intervals: telegraph, telephone, etc.? Is it reliable?

10. What is the best means of keeping track of the team's location, i.e., every other day messages to the province's health representative, an assistant appointed by the counterpart who keeps a running tally and relays information to us?

11. Determine the best means of transferring money to teams in the field, i.e., Bank Bumi Daya branches along travel route since money could be predeposited before the team ever got there.

12. In Ambon, Sulawesi, and Kalimantan, two vehicles and drivers will be needed in each province, roughly three weeks use. Can they be gotten from the province's health representative (at what price), or on the open market (compare prices)? Establish who will supply them and at what firm price during this visit. The vehicles must be in good condition, and the cost of repair during their use will be deducted from rental charge.

13. Where boats, planes, or trains are needed, get time schedules.

Basic Decisions, Staffing, and Orientation

After completion of preliminary visits to the province, project officers made three basic decisions:

1. Drawing and shipping blood was not practical, and these plans were dropped from Study IV.

2. To guard against possible loss of data shipped to Bandung by the Study IV teams, Indonesian planners devised a duplicate response column for all forms on which data could be copied. Equipped with a perforation, this duplicate column could be easily torn from the form and shipped in separate packets to Bandung.

3. Bank transfer seemed to be a practical method for delivering funds to the team leaders.

Obtaining three qualified nutritionists for the study was no real problem in view of Tarwotjo's far-flung connections in the Indonesian world of nutritionists. The decision to eliminate blood sampling from the study, plus increased recognition that vehicles would be crowded with team members and their equipment, and budgetary pressures, led to a decision to decrease the number of enumerators on each team from six to five. Because the USAID-financed jeeps had not yet been shipped from the United States, there was as yet no need for drivers. Indonesian project officers found it difficult to conceive of women participating under the hardship conditions of Study IV, so during July the project advertised for three male nurses and 15 enumerators. A total of 89 responded. These were reduced to three male nurses and 30 enumerators after a written exam and interviews. The 30 enumerators were put on half pay during training, after which 15 were finally selected.

By the end of August, the three teams had completed their classroom training and were taken to the village of Karoya in vehicles rented with HKI funds. Karoya appeared ideal as the field training site, because local officials were disappointed that they had been dropped from the second round of Study I clinical examinations. In Karoya, the three teams worked separately, each under the observation and guidance of a project officer, but in close enough proximity so that Tarwotjo could visit all three teams during the course of a day. Several locally hired horse carts stood by to transport the teams and equipment from site to site and to and from their temporary living quarters.

After a week of field training, members of the three teams went to their respective homes for two weeks of holiday. This period included the two-day annual Muslim festivities of Lebaran. On September 26, they returned to Cicendo for more conferences, to sort out their equipment and forms, receive their pay, and make other last minute preparations for their long adventure.

On September 28, the project signed a contract with a Bandung transportation firm to furnish a total of six vehicles for the three teams pending arrival of the USAID-supplied jeeps. The contract was all inclusive. Though the firm usually did not insure its vehicles, it considered insurance necessary for these distant operations. They also insisted on using company drivers and three additional driver-mechanics, one of whom was the chief mechanic of the firm. The contract also included the costs of all ferry services wherever necessary. It was also understood that where four-wheel drive vehicles were required, the contract vehicles would be traded temporarily for Jeeps or Land Rovers belonging to the provincial representative of the Health Department.

On the evening of September 29, the project held an outdoor dinner party at the house of Dr. Sommer, the American project scientist. About 70 project personnel attended. The Sommer children's dancing teacher performed with a female partner, with Javanese music piped from the Sommers' record player through a hastily assembled public address system. The West Java representative of the Health Department delivered a speech, and project personnel insisted that the two Americans also make speeches in Indonesian. The Study I team performed a skit, in which they portrayed the humorous side of interviewing parents and examining obstreperous children. The skit included appearance on the scene of a very funny, bespectacled, American-looking physician who shook hands with everyone, snapped his camera several times, and waved goodbye. The Study II and IV teams sang songs; then there was food. It was a happy occasion, commemorating one year of project operations and providing a rousing send-off for the Study IV teams.

Some months previously, project planners had discussed the seasonal dietary patterns which existed in most of Indonesia, a predominantly Muslim country. In 1977, the fasting month when most Muslims do not eat between sunrise and sunset, occurred from mid-August to mid-September. September 15-16 was the two day celebration of Lebaran, when most Muslim families visit their relatives and friends and consume extraordinary amounts of good food, enough so that food prices rise every year just prior to Lebaran. Since the sample survey would examine children only once, a true picture of the geographic distribution of vitamin A deficiency was possible only if the survey avoided inclusion of this seasonal variation in diet patterns. Thus it had long been decided that all three teams would start in Bali, where practically the entire population is Hindu. According to the 1975 Statistical Yearbook of Indonesia, Bali's population totaled 2,120,000 of whom 1,978,000 were Hindu, only 108,000 were Muslim, and 14,000 were Buddhist.

On September 30, accompanied by Tarwotjo, Djoko, and Tito, the three teams set off in six vehicles for Jogjakarta, the first leg of the journey to Bali. Anxious to arrive in Jogja before the television showing of the Mohammad Ali fight with Ernie Shavers, they left Bandung at 5:00 A.M.

PROBLEMS AND CONCLUSIONS IN BALI AND LOMBOK

Bali and Lombok were good places to begin Study IV since the islands were small enough so the teams could meet every evening to discuss their problems and standardize their operations. Standardization is important in a scientific survey. It was important that all three physicians diagnose the various abnormalities in exactly the same way and that all scales be balanced accurately. The project scientist flew to Bali and spent the first week with the three teams.

After a Monday morning meeting on October 3 with staff of the Bali representative of the Health Department, the teams set about their work. They very early showed evidence of good preparation; by the third day each team was examining 120 children.

Problems

Despite the exhaustive nature of plans and training based on the Study I experience in Java, several problems arose as a result of unique Bali circumstances:

1. Communications between the counterpart and the local authorities were inadequate, and the people had inaccurate information regarding the day of the team's arrival.

2. It was desired that initial interviews take place in the families' homes. Despite this general rule, local authorities tended to collect the families in advance at a central point. To counteract this tendency, the project sent another letter to all counterparts emphasizing that everyone in the sample area must remain at home until requested to proceed to the CP.

3. The lowest level administrative structure was the banjar. The banjar's head usually insisted that the CP be located in its main meeting hall, a large, roofed pavilion. While a convenient place for the team to work, this pavilion often was located at either end of the banjar rather than in a central location. As the banjars tended to be strung out along a road, parents sometimes had to carry their children as far as two km to the CP. Two methods were used to overcome this difficulty: first, the teams tried to arrange for location of the CP in a central location whether or not it happened to be the main meeting hall; second, they sent the team's two rented vehicles up and down the main road to pick up mothers and children on their way to the CP.

4. For the first time the project was forced to use interpreters, because most of the local inhabitants spoke only Balinese. All team members had to work through interpreters. As noted in many technical assistance projects around the world, the interpreters found it easier to answer the question directly rather than to interpret questions and answers. The enumerators were told they must insist on translation of their questions and the answers, and they should accept no questions supplied directly by the interpreter. A related problem was that the interpreter sometimes refused to work as late as the teams found it necessary.

5. Calculating the correct age in months of Balinese children proved to be impossible. Balinese used three separate calendars, none equivalent to either the Latin or Arabic calendar. The enumerators were given a Balinese calendar containing seven months of 35 days each, from which they roughly calculated the children's age in completed years. The month columns on the form were ignored except where the actual age in months was known.

6. Children less than 42 days of age were not expected to be brought to the CP. Traditionally children are kept indoors until their 42nd day, which is considered a major holiday and turning point in their life.

7. The limiting factor in speed of operation was the completion of diet interviews for random sample families. As there was no way to accelerate the process, random samples were reduced from 25% to 20%.

8. The ferry required to transport vehicles from Bali to Lombok was in dry dock. The teams, therefore, left their rented vehicles in Bali and took a passenger ferry to Lombok where they rented additional vehicles. They returned as they completed their survey of scheduled sample sites. However, the return ferry did not work every day. One team, completing its rounds on Lombok, flew all members to Surabaya in East Java where they awaited the other teams; they then cabled Bandung that they had run out of money.

Budgetary Difficulties

Project headquarters staff, Tarwotjo, Tito, and Sommer, needed to meet again with the three teams after completion of the sample sites in Bali and Lombok. For this purpose, they scheduled all teams to meet in Surabaya at the eastern end of Java on October 31. Sommer went ahead and bought his tickets, but there was a problem on the Indonesian government's part. Budgeters had considered that no supervisory trips were necessary in Java because the project was headquartered in Java. In this case, Fritz was unwilling to use HKI funds, and luckily somehow Indonesian funds became available just in time. How was this possible? Previously, Indonesian government officers had said that Central Planning Agency approval fixed the overall budgetary limits of the project; now when asked, they said there was some flexibility. However, budgetary increases had to be negotiated with other units of the department because the overall budget of the department was fixed. Project backstop officers in the department had been successful in such negotiations.

The problem of paying the vehicle contractor remained. On October 31, while in Jakarta preparing for the trip to Surabaya, Tito telephoned Fritz in Bandung to ask for the project account number. National Institute officers needed to know how to transfer funds to the project, because Tito had just picked up the check at USAID, one month after signature of the agreement.

Per Diem and Staff Difficulties

From the beginning, the Study IV teams appeared to have high morale. However, from time to time they raised questions which compared their lot in life unfavorably with that of the Study I team. The Study I team traveled each day to the field from plain but comparably comfortable headquarters in Purwakarta. They spent roughly 18 days in the field each month and received from the Indonesian government per diem for 18 days, the maximum allowed.

The Study IV teams, however, had no chance to rest and recuperate each weekend. They worked six days a week and were constantly traveling. They worried about their health. They received only 18 days per diem for a continuous 30 days in the field, and often the provincial counterparts arranged lodging where costs exceeded the per diem received. Occasionally, the teams refused to accept such accommodations, and the project found itself faced with cancellation charges.

Six months earlier, during a visit to Bandung by Health Department budgeters, Fritz had questioned the regulation concerning the maximum per diem of 18 days per month to see if there was an exception to cover people in geological surveys, for example, who had to spend long periods in the field. The truth came out; yes, there were such exceptions, but it was now too late. The budget had been prepared on the basis of the 18-day regulation, and the budget was now frozen.

Project supervisors had faced the issue squarely when confronting Study IV team members. The regulation was not a fault of the project; it was a standard government regulation. The project budget was frozen; however, there was a loophole. The budget was based upon completion of the survey at the end of May 1978 and they had been hired for the same period. If the teams could adhere to their schedule, however, they could complete the survey in late April. They would then get a one-month paid vacation, although the physicians and nutritionists would have to spend part of that time at project headquarters.

While accepting this logic when presented, the team leaders again raised the problem in a letter received at project headquarters on November 1. The letter was signed by all three team leaders. If there was to be no relief on per diem or the heavy schedule followed, then some financial allowance had to be made for occasional rest and relaxation; otherwise, the work would suffer.

Project officers in Bandung were not sure whether the letter was intended as a complaint or a veiled threat. They thought, however, that the situation was serious. Realizing that the teams that very day were meeting with Tarwotjo, Tito, and Sommer in Surabaya, project headquarters anxiously awaited their return to Bandung the following week for news of what had transpired.

Returning project officers reported that the teams were performing splendidly, they were on schedule, everyone was in good spirits, and morale was high. Per diem did not seem to be a special problem. On some occasions the teams had persuaded local officials to provide free food and lodging. Some team members had run out of money because they had spent advance per diem on Bali souvenirs.

One ophthalmologist seemed depressed, so project officers juggled schedules so he could be near his family for a week. He wired Bandung requesting that the original schedule be restored.

Conclusions

It was possible to make preliminary judgments about the prevalence of childhood eye disease. It appeared that Bali and East Java were similar to West Java, but that Lombok was much worse. The incidence of Bitot's spots ranged up to 10% in the Lombok study sites, and four cases of active corneal disease were found in 2,000 children, but no cases were found of old corneal scars. This latter fact tended to confirm earlier suspicions that children died after becoming blind. Were their deaths caused solely by disease and the depletion of nutrients, or were they in part caused by parental neglect of blind children who added a burden to families who were already poor and had all the children they needed? These questions remained to be determined.

Jeeps and Other Problems

Foreign advisors are sometimes useful in ways that have nothing to do with technical expertise. This is illustrated by Fritz's participation in the Customs clearance of the six jeeps which finally arrived in Jakarta's port on October 31, 1977. The experiences of other projects indicated that customs clearances could be a long drawn-out process. For that reason, Tito and Fritz had met earlier with the Health Department Bureau of Logistics to assure that advance preparations were made to ease and speed up the process. During the first weeks of November, the clearing agents assured Tito that everything was in order for speedy clearance. When visiting the port on Saturday, November 19, however, Tito was told that the process had become bogged down because of a change in customs personnel. A follow-up telephone call on November 22 confirmed this was still true.

In the early morning of November 23, Tito and Fritz set out for Jakarta. Arriving at the port at 9:30, they completed the administrative procedures for obtaining the requisite entry passes, then went to the agent's office. Recalling their earlier experiences at Halim, they were pleased to see large signs prominently displayed, "Do not pay 'extras' in any form whatsoever." Greeted cordially by a supervisory agent, they went to a Customs building where they arranged for another visitor's pass, then passed on to a succession of several agents who accompanied them to several Customs buildings. At each stop, they were asked to take a seat while the agent went about his work. He was seen showing the pass of the visitors from Bandung, one with an unmistakable foreign name. The clerk quickly reviewed the documents, then invited the agent into the office of the section head as soon as the previous visitor departed. Returning shortly with the required signature, the agent took his visitors to the next stop in the process. Answering Fritz's query on the smoothness of the operation, Tito remarked that the section heads preferred to sign the documents than to keep a foreigner waiting. All clearances were completed by noon. Further visits that afternoon with the Health Department Bureau of Logistics, the local jeep dealer, and USAID laid the groundwork for turning the jeeps over to the project the following week.

By this time the three Study IV teams were working in Central Java. Exchanging their rented vehicles for the jeeps, they had plenty of experience with the new vehicles by the time they arrived in Bandung for consultation just prior to the scheduled Christmas vacation. After the vacation, the teams were scheduled to complete their work in West Java. Then two of the teams would ferry four jeeps to Sumatra, a very large island west of Java where they would work for several months. The ferrying of jeeps to the other Outer Islands was too expensive and time-consuming, and therefore, was out of the question. Thus, the third team scheduled to work in Ambon, Sulawesi, and Kalimantan (Borneo) would borrow vehicles from the local Health Department representative to the extent possible; otherwise, they would resort to rental of vehicles.

The team members had been crowded in the jeeps because they had to share space with their equipment and supplies. Because of the distance from Bandung headquarters to sample sites in Sumatra, they would have to transport more equipment and supplies. The project, therefore, got the Health Department to finance the installation of roof-top luggage racks.

Another problem was ventilation. The rear section, where most team members sat, was equipped with windows which would not open. Since this was the rainy season, those in the front frequently found it necessary to close their windows, but this left the rear passengers in a heated, suffocating space. The Family Planning people had already discovered this problem and had solved it by replacing the fixed windows with two panes which could slide back and forth. The project tried to copy this innovation; however, after obtaining cost estimates, they dropped this proposed improvement.

Study I experience with its borrowed jeep indicated that some spare parts were needed from time to time. These parts would be needed for the two teams scheduled to sail to Sumatra on January 9. On December 22, Fritz called USAID to request information on the delivery of spare parts. The reply he received was that they had been delivered with the jeeps, and much discussion ensued. Half an hour later the lady called back to say that the American manufacturer expected to ship the spare parts on January 24. Asked whether this shipment would be by air or sea the lady had no information. Despite the lengthy lead time provided, it was obvious that Study IV would get very little use, if any, out of the spare parts. As it turned out, Study IV teams finished using the jeeps before the spare parts arrived.

Per Diem Problem: Resolution

On January 4, the three Study IV teams, after a well-earned Christmas leave, went with Tarwotjo and Sommer to the Sukabumi area of West Java for two days of restandardization exercises. On their return to Bandung, Tarwotjo entered into conversation with Sommer, Fritz, and Dr. Susan Pettiss, the HKI Director of Blindness Prevention who was visiting from New York. Tarwotjo reported that there was a serious morale problem: the three team leaders had calculated the Saturdays and Sundays they would spend in the field during the course of the survey; they came to a full 60 days; and they, therefore, wanted to be assured of an additional two months of pay. The team leaders wanted an answer before leaving Bandung on January 7.

The demand was an understandable one. The teams were getting the maximum of 18 days per month per diem allowed by the Health Department budgeters, but from now until the end of April they would be in continuously traveling. After a morning of budget analysis, the HKI representatives agreed once again that they could permit Study IV members to have one month of paid vacation if they adhered to their tight schedule. Only at this stage did Tarwotjo reveal that Tito and he had been analysing the Indonesian per diem budget also. They thought they could continue the per diem payment through June, an additional two months, or 36 days.

Additional Costs

On January 20, Dr. Edi called from Ambon. His team, operating with rented vehicles, had completed Ambon and was ready to fly to Manado in North Sulawesi. A slight problem had arisen, however; all planes to Manado were booked for the next week, and the only solution was to fly the team to Manado by an indirect route, thereby doubling the cost.

Why weren't the team's reservations made in advance? It seems the local counterpart was a bit cautious. He wasn't sure the team would complete its work on schedule and, therefore, held off until he was sure. Counterparts thereafter were advised to book air reservations on schedule; if need be, they could cancel them.

Repairs.

On January 30, Dr. Slamet called from Padang in Sumatra. One of his jeeps was laid up for five days for repair. He would continue working with one jeep in the meantime, but he needed Rupiah 75,000 (about $180) to cover the repair bills. The money was sent immediately. On February 2, however, Djoko received another call from Dr. Slamet. The local dealer did not have the parts required, and Slamet had sent Bandung project headquarters a list. Hopefully the list would arrive before the weekend. Djoko would take it to Jakarta, where he would meet Tito and Tarwotjo who were scheduled to arrive there on Saturday from their supervisory trip to Sulawesi. Assuming they were able to purchase the parts, they would take them to Padang on Monday. They had scheduled a supervisory trip in any case.

Air transportation.

Air was the mandatory way to travel in Sulawesi.

> The Trans-Sulawesi highway, planned to link Bitung in the north to Ujungpandang in the south, is now being intensively carried out in stages.... the highway network would stretch some 2,500 kilometers.... some 700 to 800 kilometers... would be in the form of roads to be built from scratch, and over big rivers without any bridges spanning them as yet. (2)

Dr. Sommer flew from Jakarta to Ujungpandang on January 29. He was hoping to go on to Manado the same day to meet Dr. Edi's team. However, the flight from Ujungpandang had been canceled because of bad weather. Not wanting to pay Dr. Sommer's overnight hotel bill in Ujungpandang, the airline proposed to fly him back to Jakarta on their return flight and bring him back the next day. Remembering the hazardous landing he had just experienced, Al declined this courtesy and stayed in Ujungpandang overnight.

The next day, Monday, hoping to observe Dr. Edi's team in action in the field, Al proceeded to Manado, North Sulawesi. When he arrived, he found the team had already completed its field work in the area. In fact, half of the team was waiting for a plane to Palu, because they were only able to get half of the team on the Tuesday flight, and they had booked the other half on the Monday flight. In order to make this schedule, they had worked extra hours on Friday, Saturday and Sunday. But the first contingent didn't get on its Monday flight; the plane was commandeered by an anticorruption team from Jakarta. So Al talked with the team until Tuesday and then flew back to Jakarta. Later, Tito and Tarwotjo joined the team in Palu, where they remained for the rest of the week. On the weekend Tarwotjo and Tito met Djoko in Jakarta. Since Tarwotjo had to remain in Jakarta the following week for some meetings, Djoko and Tito proceeded to Sumatra with the jeep parts.

Budget reallocations.

All of this travel, with little time left for business in Jakarta, led indirectly to money problems for the Study I team. The general pattern for securing government per diem funds was to prove first that per diem had been disbursed the previous month. This Tito generally did during his last weekend visit to Jakarta of each month. The next weekend he actually collected the money. In order to simplify an otherwise disorderly procedure, the project had been "borrowing" HKI funds to transfer per diem to the Study IV teams along with their HKI incentive pay at the first of every month. The account was repaid after receipt of government per diem funds.

On February 6, Dr. Hussaini, Study I ophthalmologist, showed up at project headquarters in Bandung. After an unsuccessful discussion with the finance officer, Hussaini approached Fritz. He had bills on his table in Purwakarta for over Rupiah 1 million ($2,500). He had to buy food for his team. He did not mention that his enumerators had to pay their monthly installment on the bank loan he had arranged for them to purchase motorcycles, but this may have been on his mind. Fritz, Soemantri, and Hussaini discussed the matter. Fritz thought Tito had probably collected the funds on Saturday and given them to Tarwotjo, who would be in Bandung later in the week. Soemantri only had a little over a million rupiah balance in the HKI account, and he thought it prudent that he only advance Hussaini half a million (about $1,200). Fritz agreed. Soemantri was right. When Tarwotjo arrived, he said Tito must have taken the funds with him to Sumatra, but when Fritz saw Tito the following week, he admitted he had not yet received the funds. He was hoping to get them the following weekend, but the following weekend they still weren't ready. There was only one weekend left in February.

Travel deterrents

Dr. Edi called Bandung from Sulawesi on February 21. The next sample site on his Central Sulawesi schedule was proving rather difficult. There was no road, and the only way to go was by a four-day horseback trek. The main trouble, though, was that ten days were required to arrange for all the horses. With a smile Tarwotjo gave his consent to deletion of this site from the schedule. But Dr. Edi had another complaint. The team was required to examine 120 children at every sample site. If there were not 120 children, they were supposed to go into the adjacent area until they examined the required number. But at Uekambuo, where they had to walk uphill for 13 Km in the rain, there were only 59 children, and the nearest other inhabited area was four Km away.

During March 1978, the two teams working in Sumatra sent their jeeps back to Bandung and flew to Kalimantan (Borneo). The project then returned the vehicles it had borrowed from USAID in Jakarta, UNICEF, and the West Java Health Service. The teams working in Kalimantan traveled by air, boat, and rented vehicles.

The walikota (mayor) of one Kalimantan town wanted to treat Dr. Slamet's team to lunch prior to their departure. The team purchased their air tickets for Pontianak, their next stop, and proceeded to the restaurant. They waited and waited, and finally the walikota showed up. Unfortunately, by the time they finished eating and arrived at the airport, their plane had taken off. The worst of it was that there was only one flight a week to Pontianak, so the team paid its cancellation charges, and took the next flight to Jakarta from where they flew to Pontianak. The team's politeness in awaiting the walikota thus proved somewhat costly.

Dreams.

One day in April, a young lady showed up at project headquarters in Bandung. She was very excited and wanted to know what had happened to her husband, a Study IV enumerator working in Kalimantan. After she calmed down, she related her previous night's dream in which her husband had appeared before her dressed in a long white gown. Tito then remembered a previous conversation with the husband. His mother had died some years previously in Kalimantan and had been buried there. He had hoped to have an opportunity to visit her grave while in Kalimantan. Given the chance, he would open his mother's grave and bring her bones back to Java. As it turned out, that's what he had been doing the previous evening.

9 The Foreign Advisor: Roles and Experiences

PERSONAL AND FAMILY CONSIDERATIONS

> We have too long focused on and debated the attributes of individuals for technical assistance, when it would be more productive to gain an understanding of the circumstances in which technical assistants work. (1)

In his review of seven different studies of Americans overseas, Francis C. Byrnes defined role shock as "... the frustrations and stresses associated with such discrepancies as between what a technical assistant views as the ideal role for himself and what he learns or finds the actual role to be abroad." He found that the American professionals seemed to take social and personal living conditions in stride, but that professional roles and relationships were a problem. Also, several of them had little understanding of administrative problems.

The key role of Dr. Alfred Sommer in the development and conduct of this project has been told to some extent in preceding chapters. The project was indeed fortunate in procuring his services. Though not yet 34 years old at the beginning of the project, he had already acquired well-earned international recognition for his epidemiological work in Bangladesh, and he brought with him rich research experiences in xerophthalmia and keratomalacia gained from surveys in El Salvador, Haiti, and previous visits to Indonesia. He was an ophthalmologic surgeon as well as an epidemiologist, and there was no one in the project who could compete with his statistical talents or his energy. He also had published widely.

While the role and contribution of Dr. Sommer as project scientist seemed assured from the outset, the role of the HKI liaison officer was less certain. In essence, this person was expected to relieve the project scientist of administrative and financial burdens and represent the interests of HKI in the project. An American living in Jakarta performed many difficult administrative chores during the early months of the project, but was unable to move to Bandung and became unavailable on a full-time basis after the beginning of 1977. HKI had based its AID contract budget on recruitment of a liaison officer in Indonesia, allowing no costs for transportation of family and household effects from the United States. Unable to recruit another American in Indonesia, HKI was haunted by this fact when they later claimed reimbursement for these costs.

HKI located the author of this case study during October 1976. Fritz, a senior AID program planner, was seeking an overseas development position to take advantage of the early Foreign Service retirement opportunity. Such retirement, on partial pension, was available to 50-year-old Foreign Service employees who had served 25 years. Fritz was 53 and could add to his 25 years of Foreign Service employment three years of World War II military service plus a year of unused sick leave.

Fritz had enjoyed a fruitful career with AID and the predecessor foreign aid agencies, probably attaining as great a sense of accomplishment as possible in any career. His motivations for an early retirement were threefold.

1. The first motivation was financial. Executive salaries had been frozen by Presidential Congressional action during recent years. On the other hand, AID was encouraging early foreign service retirements, and retirement pensions were increasing semiannually in accordance with the cost of living. Fritz gambled that his salary would not be increased. (Two months after retiring, his previous salary was increased by $8,000.)

2. Looming seven years in the future was the mandatory Foreign Service retirement age of 60. Anticipating difficulties in finding a new job at that age, Fritz had best prove now that he could do something other than government work. After joining the Indonesian project in January 1977, he learned in mid-year that the court had declared the mandatory retirement age to be unconstitutional.

3. Finally, the agency seemed increasingly bent on a suicidal course. Repeated attempts by new administrations and administrators to place their unique stamp on the agency had led to continuous reviews and revisions of policies, procedures, the scope of responsibility, and the work force by AID and outside task forces. Each review and every change was accompanied by agency pronouncements of far-reaching improvements in program content and efficiency. Indeed, these reviews left their mark on the agency, but the results were unmistakably to the agency's detriment. Both the client countries and the United States Congress became increasingly cynical, and AID's own employees, increasingly bogged down in paperwork, lost the idealism and dedication of the earlier days. Though Fritz was going to miss his old colleagues, AID seemed like a good place to leave in 1976.

It is only honest to admit that technical assistance practitioners undergo certain hardships. These hardships are recompensed not by the housing allowance or tax exemptions, but by the rewards of unusual accomplishment which accompany a technical assistance venture.

The author has experienced amoebic dysentery six times during his overseas career, thus raising life insurance costs. His children have suffered from amoebic and bacillary dysentry, diphtheria, worms, skin diseases, psychological problems, and fevers of unknown origin. One child's development was particularly worrisome; the problem was defined years later by an American psychologist as dyslexia, an educational condition untreated because it was undiagnosed.

Overseas practitioners sometimes sell houses at a loss before an urgent overseas departure. Household goods are broken en route and must be replaced at higher prices. Appliances remain in storage, as they are unusable at some overseas posts; upon returning to the United States, one finds them in a deteriorated condition. Electric motors are repeatedly jammed and finally discarded after alternating use between 50 and 60 cycle current, and the curtains of the last house never fit the windows of the next house. These are facts ignored by those who seek to tax the fringe benefits of overseas workers.

Problems usually begin when the practitioner makes his decision to take the overseas job. When Dr. Sommer accepted the Indonesian position in the spring of 1976, he was an Ophthalmology Fellow at the Wilmer Institute of the Johns Hopkins Hospital in Baltimore. After he rented out his house and stored his family effects, HKI sent him with his wife and two children to the Netherlands where they studied Indonesian and awaited receipt of formal government clearance, along with approval of their long-term visa applications. Meanwhile, the

HKI finance officer, Al Lisi, was awaiting the same clearances in New York. Planning a trip to Jakarta to set up the project accounts, he finally went in the absence of formal clearances. Perhaps he could help speed them up.

Living out of suitcases for a lengthy period is never much fun under the best of circumstances. Added to this were the worries about the project and entering the Sommer children in the Bandung school on September 1. And the only word from Jakarta was that government clearances had become bogged down, Tito was hurt in an auto accident, and Tarwotjo appeared to be abandoning ship. By August 1, the Sommers were on pins and needles: what could be more disheartening after severing secure ties with the past? Did the Indonesians want to do the project, or didn't they?

At this point Dr. Sommer's thoughts flashed back to previous Indonesian visits, and he wondered what they portended for the future, assuming that the project was finally approved. He knew that official red tape could be frustrating, and he recalled his previous summer in Indonesia. At that time, in order to get official permission to visit rural areas, he had turned over to the Indonesian Cabinet Secretariat (SEKKAB) his passport along with a dozen pictures and numerous forms which had to be revised several times. He then proceeded on field trips with his Indonesian colleagues. Two months later, permission still had not been granted. In order to leave Indonesia, he asked Tarwotjo to collect his passport, explaining he had changed his mind and would not be visiting rural areas. He had been able to get away with this as an individual on a short-term assignment, but such procedures were impossible when the project needed to send dozens of people around the countryside to number houses and collect data.

Learning of a BAPPENAS (Indonesian planning agency) meeting scheduled for August 29 which might result in project clearances, but recognizing this would not lead to immediate visa clearances, the Sommers decided to apply for visitor visas. At the Indonesian Embassy, they learned they could get a four-week visa within two or three days. However, they happened upon a cable, correctly addressed but misdirected to the wrong hotel. This cable, sent by the HKI finance officer from Jakarta, advised them to remain where they were.

August 17 was a frustrating day. Hoping for a night stopover in Iran, the only one possible, the Sommers boarded a train for The Hague and a taxi to the Iran Embassy where they applied for Iranian visas. Everything went well until the consular official attempted to stamp visas in the Sommer passports. The Sommers, international travelers as they were, had no empty pages remaining in their passports and had to return to the American Consulate in Amsterdam.

The next day, August 18, while Mrs. Sommer was taking the new United States passport to the Iranian Embassy, Dr. Sommer received a phone call from the HKI finance officer in Jakarta. The latter was expecting to meet with BAPPENAS and SEKKAB the following day, August 19. Hopefully they would cable the Sommer visas on Saturday. Once the visas were assured, the Sommers could book their Pan Am flight, but it looked increasingly as if there would be no overlap in Jakarta with Al Lisi, now scheduled to depart on August 28.

On Friday, August 20, the Indonesian Embassy phoned. The Sommer visa clearances had arrived, and the family should come to the Embassy on Monday, August 23, to fill out forms. Dr. Sommer asked if there was any chance they could receive their visas the same day. The consular officer laughed and asked why Dr. Sommer was always in a hurry -- his previous visits and calls had apparently gained him a reputation -- since these things always take two or three days.

Om Monday morning, after a train trip from Amsterdam, the Sommer family arrived at the Embassy doorstep as it opened for business. A Hollander preceding them advised he had an "in"; having submitted his passport on Friday he would receive it back this morning. Surprise of surprises, however, he was told by the man at the desk that the "visa man" had gone on vacation and should be back in "a few days." This seemed an inauspicious beginning. Dr. Sommer went to the head of the line, nevertheless, and told his story. He received the identical response. After Al blew his top, the man scurried away to find the officer who had asked them to come on Monday. The visas were ready that afternoon.

For those who are not aware of it, employees of agencies under contract with AID must travel by American carrier unless there's definite, provable inconvenience, such as none being available. For the Sommers, who preferred not to have to prove the inconvenience, this meant they had to fly Pan Am to Hong Kong, then take the once weekly Pan Am flight to Jakarta. A person not traveling with these restrictions would have done the sensible thing, fly to Bangkok or Singapore and take one of the many flights of other airlines on a daily basis to Jakarta.

Hong Kong is a long way from Amsterdam, and the only place Pan Am landed in time for an overnight rest was Teheran. Hoping to arrange such a stop while awaiting the visas, Al took the train back to Amsterdam and hurried off to Pan Am. He was able to get the family on a flight to Teheran the very next morning. However, they would have to stop over for two nights at airline expense because no space was available on the next flight out of Teheran.

Without an identifying passport, Al was unable to cash travelers checks at a bank to pay his bills, so he went to American Express, then back by train to the Hague for the passports with signed visas. The Sommers made it to the airport the following morning, and they made it to Jakarta on Saturday, August 28, missing the HKI finance officer by a half day, but greeted warmly by Tarwotjo, Tito, and Dan Goldsmith, a short-termer on the project. BAPPENAS approval of the project had been cabled to HKI in New York the previous day.

Though the agreement was signed within a few days, nothing much else happened. Tito had emerged from his hospitalization, but Dr. Sugana's back problem continued, and Tarwotjo, remaining in Jakarta, sounded increasingly like he was unavailable for the project. Several other key professionals previously expected to participate were no longer available, and three decision making officers of the Department of Health were out of the country. Moreover, there was no office furniture, typewriters, or clerical staff. The first month was spent looking for a house in Bandung, getting the children enrolled in school, visiting the local Immigration Office, reviewing project budgets, commiserating with Dr. Sugana at his bedside, and traveling to Jakarta to expedite project arrangements with the Department of Health, other Indonesian government offices, WHO, UNICEF, and USAID, and making arrangements to purchase a locally assembled automobile.

Logistics Problems

Foreigners working in a strange country encounter what are euphemistically referred to as "logistical problems": how do personnel straighten out their affairs with the Immigration Department and the local police; how do they arrange for Customs clearance and local transport of personal and professional effects; how do they find and lease a house, register their car, and obtain a driver license; where do they send their children to school; and what allowances are provided? A newcomer to overseas technical assistance assumes he will spend his time abroad using his professional knowledge and skills for the benefit of the host country. Oldtimers know that a large proportion of the time is frequently spent on administrative and logistical problems.

Previous Arrangements

Formerly, AID missions were staffed to assist in the process. Their staff included indigenous personnel, who through long experience became skilled in these logistical processes. Well-known to local airport, harbor, immigration, police, and Customs authorities, they could move quickly and skillfully in these circles. It was not necessary for AID contractor personnel in most cases to put in an appearance to get these jobs done. Over the years, succeeding United States administrations perceived that the size of their overseas missions were harmful to American foreign policy interests. They increasingly called for lowering the American "profile." One way in which AID supposedly achieved this objective was by eliminating logistical support of its overseas contractors. The first result was the premature retirement or outright firing of hundreds of previously loyal employees of the United States Government through large "reduction-in-force" programs. The second result was the entry of hundreds of Americans into local government offices where they previously had never been seen and under frustrating circumstances where they were the most unsuitable representatives possible of American foreign policy interests.

Large contractors with large multi-year contracts may ease the situation by hiring indigenous personnel to assist in these logistical processes, but many small contractors like HKI have no choice but to charge their American employees with their own logistical support.

Visas

As a former long-term AID employee, Fritz had his original exposure to the process when he applied for a visa at the Indonesian Embassy in Washington during November 1976. When asked about his expected length of stay in Indonesia, Fritz responded that he hoped to stay for two and a half years on an Indonesian government project. This response determined the application form he was given. It was an extremely long form to be completed with four copies. After reviewing the application which required the names, addresses and dates for the high school and four universities he attended, the consular officer requested that Fritz also list his elementary school. Though no space remained for this purpose, he was asked to "just squeeze it in."

After a subsequent interval, the consular officer returned and said they could expect Jakarta approval within six months. Fritz argued that this was an impossible situation. He was expected to be in Indonesia by January 1. Oh, in that case, Mr. Fritz should fill out the visitor's application. A visitor's visa was good for a few days, but Fritz could apply for a permanent visa upon his arrival. Fritz noted with some alarm that in filling out the form he was promising to leave Indonesia after a few days and that any falsehood would be fully prosecuted.

A family situation complicated matters. Fritz's wife was a Thai national. Sworn in as an American citizen on December 14, she went from the United States District Court to the United States Passport

Office to apply for a passport. The next day the two of them departed for short stops in New York and Ohio. Her passport was received by mail in Ohio a few hours before departure for the airport. Mrs. Fritz still needed an Indonesian visa. Meanwhile, project staff in Indonesia had arranged for three-month clearances which the government wired to Hong Kong. Arriving there in late December, both the writer and his wife secured the longer term visas which were stamped in their passports.

Foreign Travel

The arrival of Fritz and his wife in Jakarta on January 3 was not particularly well-timed. Dr. Sommer had been awaiting the arrival of an administrative person for months, but he was scheduled for a quick trip to the United States on January 5, a date which could not be postponed. He did his best to orient Fritz with the project and his duties on January 4. On the morning of January 5, they went their separate ways with Mrs. Sommer accompanying the Fritzes in a dilapidated Holden stationwagon on the four-hour road trip from Jakarta to Bandung.

During a lifetime of world travel, Fritz had enjoyed many examples of scenic beauty. Nevertheless, he appreciated the route to Bandung which revealed breathtaking panoramas of rugged mountains, deep ravines and gorges, steep slopes of green tea, and terraced hillsides of irrigated rice. The road was blacktop asphalt but quite narrow, and many houses and shops were built disturbingly close to the road. Signs of the famed population density of Java were evident everywhere, mainly in the form of people, people, and more people.

But an automobile trip between Bandung and Jakarta can also be a perilous adventure. The road is not a highway, but Indonesian drivers act as if it were. At peak periods of traffic, vehicles of all sizes and vintages move bumper to bumper over long stretches of road, coming to a halt with each mishap, and moving again as the wreckage is shoved to the side. Drivers continually attempt to pass, swerving in and out of oncoming traffic, and squeezing between moving cars already too close for comfort. A stop to purchase fruits or vegetables from the stands at the side of the road quickly results in a traffic jam.

The narrow two-lane road winds and climbs tortuously to the Puncak, a pass at 5,500 feet elevation located halfway between Bandung and Jakarta. Except during the driest season, one expects to encounter a heavy fog for some miles on both sides of the Puncak. Oncoming cars operate with blinking emergency lights, fog lights, and spot lights. Huge buses loom out of the mist and pass with a loud continuous blast of the horn. Speeding toward you over the top of a hill or around the next sharp curve is a car on the wrong side of the road. After swerving to miss that misguided driver, the car comes to a screeching halt just behind a truck stopped at the side of the road for repairs. And one never quite escapes from the swarms of buzzing motorcycles which help to enliven the journey.

Travel on a rainy night just adds a bit more adventure. Many Indonesian drivers are of the type one often finds in Asian countries who find it unsatisfying to leave their headlights on a steady dim beam. They prefer to switch between brights and parking lights. Many just switch them off, perhaps to save the battery. In the dark spaces between the blinking lights, one strains to peer through the swinging windshield wipers to catch a glimpse of those objects which he perceives to be in the dark spaces between the blinking lights, usually unlit bicycles, horsedrawn vehicles, or children walking along the road. Neither Sommer nor Fritz took this journey more than was necessary, but it was necessary more often than would have been preferred.

Housing Arrangements

After arriving in Bandung, Fritz visited census operations in the field, studied files and reports, and acquainted himself with the nittygritty administrative details of the project. Mrs. Fritz concentrated on house-hunting, and her husband joined her on the most likely possibilities. She looked at 60 houses altogether. There were some beautiful large houses, some with swimming pools and large gardens; these were impractical for a small family. Others were impractical for other reasons. Houses without telephones were passed up because obtaining a telephone required a lengthy wait after a $2,300 installation charge. The biggest problem was the adequacy of water and electricity. They finally negotiated on a modest two-bedroom house where the government had already approved an increase in the electrical capacity to 2,000 watts. Hard bargaining finally achieved a decrease of the rent from $800 to $650 a month with the entire two and a half year lease payable in advance. The Fritzes moved into the house January 31 after cabling HKI to ship their air freight.

Required Forms and Automobile Purchases

Meanwhile, there were other logistical problems to overcome. Fingerprints were taken and forms filled out at the Bandung office of the Immigration Department. At one point, officials said a one-year residence would have to be taken up with the Jakarta office. Fortunately, the sister of the project's chief secretary was employed in the local immigration office. After the two sisters got together, somehow matters were straightened out.

The purchase of a car was not a simple matter. To stimulate the local assembly of vehicles, the government had severely restricted imports. However, its agreement with HKI permitted the American employees to purchase locally assembled vehicles free of tax. The first step was to choose an automobile which could be readily available. This was relatively easy. The next step was to apply to the Cabinet Secretariat (SEKKAB) for approval of the purchase. This was done on January 11, and approval was duly granted. After arranging for temporary registration in Jakarta, the car was picked up in early February. A host of documents came with the car, including a list of the engine and chassis numbers of all unassembled vehicles carried in the same ship with the Fritz car when delivered in Indonesia. The dealer specifically warned Fritz to hold on to all documents. He was mystified as to their usefulness, but he later learned.

Personal Possessions

Personal possessions arrived at the Jakarta international airport, Halim, on January 27. As soon as a copy of the airway bill was received, application was made to SEKKAB for duty free entry. Approval was delayed for a few days since the officer in charge was out sick. He was reportedly signing approvals from his bed, but it took him a few days to get to the Fritz application. Visiting SEKKAB on February 11, Fritz found concern about the inclusion of four television trays in the packing list. As most Americans know, these are flimsy stands on which individuals can place snacks or drinks while they watch the television programs. They also come in handy for guests who sit in comfortable chairs as they munch a buffet luncheon. But apparently "TV trays" was suspicious nomenclature for someone in SEKKAB.

From SEKKAB Fritz took the airway bill and SEKKAB approval to a building near Halim where he left the documents at 9:00 A.M. Returning for the PPUD at 3:00, Fritz went to Halim Customs where the first key officer he was to meet was out for the day. Luckily, he met an Indonesian employee of another American foundation who offered to help with clearances. He would telephone Fritz when he needed to be present. Fritz waited patiently in Bandung, then began to get anxious. Finally he received a telephone call suggesting that he appear at Halim early the morning of February 23. Although a bothersome, aggravating process, the groundwork laid made Customs clearance less difficult than the situation described in Chapter 6. It was completed prior to noon.

Then came negotiations for transport of the personal effects to Bandung. Two small trucks were required. Though Fritz argued long and hard, company officials would not budge from their first exorbitant price of $450. Company officers offered to cut the price in half if Fritz could provide a return Bandung-Jakarta load the same day. This he could not do, of course, so they packed the two trucks, which Fritz followed to Bandung in his personal car.

Arriving at Bogor, the truck drivers decided to use a new road which largely bypassed the city. A policeman approached at the entrance allowed them to proceed. As they came to the exit, however, whistles shrieked and the trucks were stopped by several policemen who took the drivers' licenses and other identity papers. The police tried to wave Fritz on, but he parked the car and tried to talk to them. At this point his command of the language was quite elementary, and he pretended he could not speak Indonesian at all. The police said the Fritz car could proceed. However, trucks from Jakarta were prohibited from using the road. Fritz wanted to know what was going to happen and how much time was required, but the police were unable to tell him. It would depend on their superiors who had not yet arrived. Fritz insisted he had to stay with the trucks until they delivered his personal effects to his house in Bandung. Finally, after an hour of standing around, the police suddenly returned the identity papers of the drivers, and the trucks were allowed to proceed to Bandung where they unloaded that night.

Obtaining a permanent car registration, driver's licenses, and identification cards required repeated visits over a period of several weeks to the Bandung Customs office, traffic police, and the municipal building. One of the hospital physicians happened to be a police officer. She and one of the project secretaries assisted the Fritzes in this seemingly never ending process.

Additional Procedures

The RT is the lowest geographical administrative unit in Indonesia and refers to a neighborhood of roughly 30-60 houses. To start the process, Fritz took his passport to the chairlady of the RT and asked for a letter attesting to his residence. The only trouble was that this lady was visiting Jakarta. After her return a week or so later, she gladly furnished the letter.

It is difficult to describe the process, because the Fritzes usually did not understand what was going on. They visited a number of offices where they found clerks checking and stamping forms. Many passport-size and smaller photos were required, as well as the original marriage certificate. It was with some surprise, then, when the Fritzes found they had to pose for another camera shot taken by the traffic police. They provided full family histories with several copies listing names, ages, occupations, and addresses of parents, in-laws, and children. In one room, they joined a large group of aspiring Indonesian drivers filling out long forms in triplicate which included nomenclature describing the shapes of their heads, ears, noses, and chins. Instructions with pictures were posted on the wall to guide the aspiring drivers.

In the midst of this process, one officer found that Fritz did not possess the original of the PPUD stamped for the police. He had several copies stamped for other offices, but none for the police and the process had to stop. Fritz called the dealer in Jakarta, who at first insisted the document was not needed, then agreed to obtain and send the document to Fritz. Describing the procedure later to a brigadier general of police who was an acquaintance in Jakarta, Fritz was told that this was a holdover from the old days. A new streamlined procedure had been installed in Jakarta, but unfortunately it had not yet been extended to Bandung. Nevertheless, the process was finally completed.

Housing and Educational Allowances

Then there was the matter of housing and educational allowances. These expenses were reimbursable under the AID-HKI contract. In a letter of September 30, 1976, the contracting officer for AID in Washington wrote HKI that these allowances were controlled by the standardized regulations for government civilians in foreign areas. In conferences with AID's contracting officers at that time, HKI was instructed to obtain a statement from USAID in Jakarta that expenses for these purposes were in line with policy and costs in Indonesia. During January and February of 1977, Fritz discussed the matter with a management officer for USAID in Jakarta who suggested that Fritz write him a letter. This Fritz did on February 23. The USAID reply of March 7 was satisfactory so far as the housing allowance was concerned. In regard to educational allowances, however, the letter stated that the allowance according to standardized regulations was $250 per year.

Such allowances are based on surveys of costs undertaken by the United States Department of State. Obviously, no survey had been made of educational costs in Bandung for some years. The Sommer children had been enrolled in a school cooperatively managed by foreigners living in the community. Tuition costs for each child amounted to $1,150. The allowance was $2,580 for Jakarta and $1,650 for Bogor. However, since the survey for Bandung was out of date, it seemed that HKI was expected to shell out an extra couple of thousand dollars per year for the education of the Sommer children, although HKI had every reason to believe when signing the AID contract that these costs would be reimbursed.

The USAID letter offered two suggestions:

1. Bring the matter to the attention of the AID contracting officer for consideration in authorizing payment of excess costs "as it may be allowed under the terms of the contract."

2. Complete an attached education allowance questionnaire "which will be used in establishing more realistic allowances for Bandung in the future."

Fritz sent USAID the completed education allowance questionnaire. He also informed HKI in New York of the contents of the USAID letter. Subsequent HKI efforts to obtain relief from AID in Washington were in vain, however, because the contracting officer continued to insist that USAID in Jakarta corroborate the claims made by HKI.

Fritz, therefore, visited the embassy's Joint Administrative Section on September 27. Embassy officers sympathized and suggested that Fritz send them a letter from the head of the Bandung school which certified actual costs. Fritz forwarded such a letter on October 10 and this letter was transferred to USAID for action. Meanwhile, the USAID management officer who had been dealing with these matters had been transferred to another country. His replacement replied to the Fritz letter as follows:

> As you are aware, the education allowance is limited to employees. In this case, we cannot identify documentation of such relationship to the Agency for International Development.
>
> You may wish to furnish the above mentioned documentation to this office for further consideration.

Patience will sometimes win the day. After receiving this response, Fritz replied with a full history of the problem and attached copies of all previous correspondence. He sighed with relief on receiving a memorandum of November 28 from USAID in Jakarta which admitted that the standardized regulations were clearly out of date and understated, confirmed that the embassy was taking action to correct the situation, and suggested that HKI might use the memo in its "appeal to the contracting officer that your claim is in line with the policy and costs in Indonesia."

One would have thought that settled the matter. However, on February 13, 1978, Fritz received a call on the hospital telephone from a new embassy personnel officer. Had he yet filled out the educational allowance forms she had sent him? Fritz indicated that as a matter of fact he hadn't yet received them, and explained he had submitted the forms a year ago. However, the new personnel officer had no knowledge of this fact. It so happened that Fritz was headed for Jakarta that very afternoon and he took the file with him. When he met the embassy officer, she was just about to take the action needed to correct the situation which Fritz thought had taken place the previous November.

CULTURAL ASPECTS

> ... it is difficult to work where there is no opportunity to check on what is understood by the counterpart. . . . (2)

Communications among the parties in a technical assistance project can be very important. Language and little cultural subtleties sometimes present obstacles to effective communications.

Culture

What is this thing called "culture" which often befuddles aid administrators and technical assistance practitioners, and how does one deal with it? A famous American author of books on Hindu and Buddhist religion and philosophy once exclaimed that a lifetime of concentrated study had not prepared him for the shock of his first visit to India.

There are many books on the subject, and overseas travelers should read those which pertain to the countries where they work. But usually they don't quite prepare a person for the intimate working relationships he experiences in a technical assistance project. And lest the reader think that only practitioners in foreign countries experience cultural problems, it may be useful to know that a major study on social change in the United States concludes that "middle class practitioners who engage with social and ethnic minorities in slum environments operate under analogous conditions of cultural distance and are faced with similar enormous problems. (3)

Every society and subsociety has a system of values, the rules of which govern the thoughts and actions of its members. These rules are not simply a matter of law or even what we refer to as custom. They refer to the way we think, talk, walk, eat, express our emotions, and treat our fellow beings in society under the whole spectrum of possible circumstance. They stem from the whole history of the society, its language, its basic philosophies, its religions, its economy, the relationship between government and the people, even the climate. We individuals learn the basic rules as children, and they become firmly embedded in our subconscious for automatic action and reaction for the remainder of our lives.

While all societies have value systems, the value systems are not the same. In the situation under discussion, the HKI representatives were fluent in English, their behavior was conditioned by lifetime immersion in a modernized, industrial society which dominated a continent characterized by sharp seasonal contrasts. Their behavior from childhood was governed by an ethic steeped in the yes-no, black-white, beginning-end confrontational attitudes of the Judaic-Christian Euro-American tradition and by living in a society with strong beliefs in cause-and-effect relationships and the ability of human beings to solve problems and to control nature.

Indonesians make their home in a widely scattered group of islands. They speak many languages, though Bahasa Indonesia is the official language and the one used for communication between speakers of two other languages. They inherit three layers of cultural patterns, the indigenous Indonesian, Hindu, and Islamic, which have been compounded together in various forms now challenged by outside modern influences. A tropical country, Indonesian development has been conditioned by the ever present volcanic mountains and the nearness of the warm Indian and Pacific Oceans. Most Indonesians still live in traditional villages, only a minority have received a meaningful education, and many still attach great value to rearing large families and living in harmony with nature and society. Throughout Indonesia aesthetic values, art, music, and traditional dancing hold important positions in present day life, a fact which helps make the stay of the technical assistance practitioner a most pleasant one.

Communications

Communications between Americans and host country personnel in a technical assistance project are not unlike communications processed through radio transmitters. Military and diplomatic organizations sometimes transmit and receive secret messages. An American wishing to send a message types it in English, then hands it to a cryptographer who types it into a machine which encodes it. When the message emerges from the encoder it is unintelligible in any language. The message is then handed to the person who transmits it.

Assuming a radio system, the operator may tap an electric key which transmits Morse signals through an electronic radio transmitter and an antenna from which the signals are carried over hundreds or thousands of miles of radio waves to their destination. Passage of these signals through electric storms serves to dim the signal and surround it with atmospheric noises. Enemy signals may jam the radio waves and distort the message. The receiver, human or machine, records the message as received, types it into the language of the encoding device, and passes it through a decoding device. Assuming the decoding device is set with the same code as the encoding device of the transmitter and every other part of the system has operated perfectly, the message is then typed in English as the message originally typed by the sender. If there are garbles, the receiving organization requests a retransmission. However, redundancy in the original message improves chances of its being understood in the first transmission.

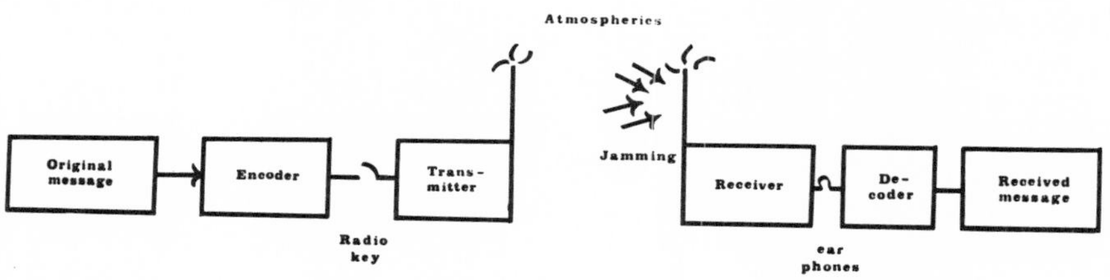

Fig. 9.1. A Communications System.

A similar communications system takes place between counterparts in a technical assistance project. The speaker thinks in his own language and transmits his message in a somewhat garbled version of the language of the receiver. The receiver understands the message to the extent he is able to decode it and determine its true intent. What were the systems of logic which formed the message in the mind of the speaker? What cultural values lay behind the message transmitted? A little redundancy may help, perhaps a repetition of the message in the language of the speaker.

Cultural Requirements

Requirements for understanding and appreciating cultural differences and local sensitivities will vary according to the role performed by the visitor, the nature of the project in which he is engaged, and the length and intensity of the cooperative relationship. A person with recognized, outstanding expertise may be forgiven for his foibles more often than the advisor with only average expertise. This person, if not sensitive to the local scene, may best be used for short-term assignments so he can complete his job before personal relations become more important than the job to be performed. A short-term consultant called in to advise on the installation and operation of equipment will have a minimum requirement. An engineer or physical scientist dealing with mathematical formulas and physical facts will likely have a lesser requirement than a person dealing with organizational structures and the analysis and interpretation of social science problems. An advisor who must await decisions on initial recommendations before proceeding to an operational phase, or one who must exert pressure on local staff to implement his recommendations, will likely encounter more sensitivity than the expert who completes his assignment with a set of drawings. The foreign advisor who works daily with his local colleagues and participates in project decision making over a two or three year period has a very high requirement. If he simultaneously exerts some control over the purse strings of the project, the requirement is maximized. Sommer and Fritz fell into this latter category.

Both Sommer and Fritz had served in other countries, had learned other languages, and had enjoyed relationships with many Hindus, Buddhists, and Muslims. They recognized the value of looking at problems from the viewpoint of others. They were probably as well equipped culturally to engage in an overseas technical assistance project as anyone. Yet they had some problems communicating with their colleagues. There were never serious conflicts, but sometimes Americans and Indonesians had difficulty in understanding each other. And although language was a problem, it was not simply a language problem. It just sometimes seemed as if they were talking past each other without being in direct communication.

> ...foreign aid tends to succeed or fail, psychologically and materially, depending on whether the aid relationship strengthens or weakens the recipients' self-esteem. (4)

Intellectual imperialism is wrong. (5)

Generally speaking, recipient government officials are fairly sensitive about technical assistance relationships. Most have a sense of national pride, and sometimes have educational qualifications which match or surpass those of the advisor. They know a chasm exists in the matter of economic development. Nevertheless, it makes them uncomfortable to read in a Western newspaper about the "backwardness" of their country or to receive lengthy sermons on the subject by a USAID mission director. They know they have problems, but they don't want the foreign expert to run them into the ground, particularly since he just arrived yesterday and will be gone tomorrow.

Many donor agency officials seem oblivious to these sensitivities. A letter from USAID in Jakarta to the Indonesian National Institute for Health Research and Development missed the principle entirely by referring to the Nutritional Blindness Prevention Project as a project conducted by HKI. Around the world USAID employees are accustomed to referring to local government projects assisted by USAID as if they were USAID projects. They do likewise in Congressional testimony read with interest by proud officials of recipient governments. After many years of cooperating with other governments, how long will it be before we begin to recognize the fact that these are not our projects? The projects belong to the host government; we assist.

In a similar vein, project documents drafted by donor government personnel sometimes refer to technical assistance advisors with such titles as Project Leader, Research Coordinator, or Chief Engineer. Every outside expert with such a title has at least one strike against him when he arrives in the host country. In the case of Al Sommer, all top project titles were determined in a meeting in Jakarta during his consultation visit in 1975. His title was to be Project Scientist. Yet all AID-HKI communications, including the contract, refer to him as the Principal Investigator.

Starting a project from scratch can offer real challenges, opportunities, and problems for the outside advisor. Recognizing the limited time frame of the project, noting that Indonesian staff did not seem to be aggressively pushing for a project start, and despite his feelings for Indonesian sensitivities, the project scientist exerted strong pressure in September 1976, and the project began to move. People were hired, furniture and equipment were purchased, funds began to flow, and project activity increased until it achieved the unstoppable momentum described in earlier chapters.

THE ROLE OF THE FOREIGN ADVISOR

> ... We are always made to feel that the foreigner is a very honored person and we are just lay persons. When we think a foreigner is a very high person and we are very low, it is not easy to be equal in the work. (6)

Generally, a technical advisor is expected by his host country colleagues to advise and consult, not to exert leadership of the activity. It is, therefore, best to let the local project leaders make the decisions, exert leadership and control of the activity, and get credit for the accomplishments.

Project Leadership

The amount of leadership exerted by Al Sommer in the project under discussion, however, was quite substantial. How was he able to get away with it, and why were there no serious repercussions? The reasons are manifold. First was the personality of Al Sommer himself, acting and interacting in tandem with the personalities of the Indonesian project leaders. Close behind was the recognized expertise and authority which he represented. Third was the nature of the project, a temporary activity with some Indonesian project leaders dividing their time between it and their other responsibilities. Finally, there was the manner by which Al Sommer demonstrated his worth and played the role of a project team member.

Dr. Sommer possessed some understanding of the aspirations of his Indonesian colleagues. Thus when Tarwotjo appeared as if he were not going to be available for the project, Sommer not only protested vigorously but also persuaded him that the project offered the most promising opportunity available for Tarwotjo to secure his Ph. D. But he didn't just suggest the possibility. He went to the rector of a local university and secured his promise to put Tarwotjo on the staff, thereby enabling him to fulfill the Ph. D. requirements without attending class.

Demonstrating considerable energy, Sommer traveled with Indonesian staff to rural clinics to obtain relevant data and to carry out the minisurvey described in Chapter 3. His previous experiences proved immediately helpful in determining what data were relevant and what information was not worth collecting. He reviewed the first draft of forms and manuals for the census survey and the Study I examinations with other members of the headquarters team, seeking their advice as well as that of accomplished Indonesian survey specialists. The Indonesian staff and Sommer worked together to iron out the special problems of asking particular kinds of questions in the local environment.

It was not Al Sommer's makeup to take a back seat in any environment. Almost always it was he who suggested to project leaders that a meeting was required, until finally they accepted the need for regularly scheduled staff sessions. Almost always it was he who put forward the agenda items, spelled out the issues, used the blackboard to elucidate his analyses of problems, and provided alternative suggestions for their solution, giving his own preference but always emphasizing that their decision was needed. Either they accepted the preferred solution, or a discussion ensued after which a decision was made.

Al Sommer was analytical, had a very quick mind, and was persuasive in his arguments. He tended to lead the Indonesian project leaders into his preferred solution. Occasionally, they raised arguments to which he listened carefully. If their arguments carried weight, he bowed to them and congratulated his colleagues for their excellent ideas. Occasionally he did not understand the arguments, but understood there were reasons in the Indonesian environment which required a different course of action than the one he advocated. Indonesians sometimes found it difficult to explain the real underlying reason that a certain course of action could not work.

The project leadership acted like a council. When the council required a chairman, the group, including Sommer, looked to Tarwotjo to play that role. Often Sommer got together in advance with Tarwotjo and/or Sugana to discuss and gain a common understanding of particular issues. A subsequent meeting with other project leaders would then lead to quicker decisions with less deliberation. But Pak Tarwotjo was not always available. Most generally he did not arrive in Bandung until Tuesday, frequently not until Wednesday. Some weeks he could not make it to Bandung at all. On such occasions, other project staff tended to look to Dr. Sommer for leadership. He did not disappoint them.

Some matters required leadership by Indonesians. Discipline, if required, had to be exerted by Tito. If professional persons were involved, Tarwotjo or Dr. Sugana had to exert it. But even in such cases, Indonesian leaders sometimes asked Sommer to participate in discussions with the offender. Confrontation is not an enjoyable experience for many Indonesians, and often they tend to avoid it. Sometimes they also chose their American colleagues to share in the onus of the situation.

Nepotism

Dr. Sommer accepted and invited this onus in connection with the nepotism which almost but not quite penetrated project operations. We Westerners must admit that nepotism is present in our world as well as in the less modern areas of the globe. On a philosophical level, however, we believe in merit and ability as the principal basis for the awarding of contracts and the appointment of personnel. In other parts of the world, personal and family relationships are far more important and are a principal means through which work objectives are sought and accomplished. The family member who succeeds in attaining an influential position is expected and pressured to take care of his relatives. If he does not do so, he loses respect in the society to which he belongs. Thus, while President Kennedy was criticized in the United States for appointing relatives to important positions, he was roundly applauded in other countries for the same reason.

So, when Al Sommer found out that the project was about to hire people related to persons already on the job, he gave a little speech in which he said that the hiring of relatives and friends was <u>verboten</u>. It was against Foundation policy, and its violation would get everybody fired. He stated that he understood the pressures to which they were subject and requested that they use him as the "fall guy." They should tell relatives that Dr. Sommer opposed their hire, or they could say that Dr. Sommer insisted on interviewing and approving all appointments personally.

Additional Tensions

During the early days of installing project headquarters in the Cicendo Eye Hospital, certain tensions developed between project and hospital personnel. These probably got out of hand because the key to their solution, Dr. Sugana, hospital director and clinical investigator for the project, was himself lying in a hospital bed with a severe back problem. During ensuing efforts to ameliorate the situation, Dr. Sommer became increasingly involved in hospital affairs. He assumed special duties, accompanying hospital ophthalmologists on teaching rounds and performing surgical operations. Frequently requested to provide consultation an special cases, he was also asked to perform emergency surgery on the assist director's grandmother. By Indonesian request he also served on a special committee to organize an

Indonesia postgraduate ophthalmology seminar. In addition, he asked hospital authorities to send him all cases of xerophthalmia which entered the hospital. While this resulted in frequent interruptions at his desk, it also provided some valuable experience for the planning and conduct of Study II.

Clinical Leadership

An enthusiastic advisor, Al Sommer's enthusiasm was sometimes infectious. Among unique cases brought to him was Simina, a 25-year-old woman reporting to a clinic in which a hospital physician worked part time. Simina appeared healthy and well nourished, but possessed the unmistakable symptoms of vitamin A deficiency, classical conjunctival and corneal xerosis. Dr. Sommer had previously theorized, like others, that such corneal changes occurred only in severely malnourished children. Simina, however, did not possess the blinding form of the disease called keratomalacia; perhaps the latter form required severe malnutrition as a causal agent.

Six days of treatment with oral vitamin A cleared Simina's condition. Hospital doctors became enthusiastic, and Dr. Sugana joined in the examinations. They took photographs of Simina's eyes and took "before and after" biopsies which Dr. Sommer sent to the Wilmer Institute at Johns Hopkins for analysis. One important aspect of the case was that Simina's retinal lesions had caused severe impairment of her visual field. Was it possible that treatment of children for corneal disease was not as helpful as previously thought? Dr. Sommer had planned to study this aspect in Study II children, but it was helpful to examine a cooperative adult rather than a screaming, wriggling child, and he got information on symptoms and visual fields as well as good retinal photographs not possible with a child.

The dietary interview clearly demonstrated the difficulty of obtaining accurate information from rural Indonesians. Dr. Sugana and Tarwotjo joined in asking the questions. What did Simina eat? Oh, she ate everything. Just exactly what did she eat? Oh, she ate rice. What else did she eat; did she eat fruit and vegetables? Yes, sometimes. How often? Oh, fairly often. Did she eat fish? Yes. Fresh fish or dried fish? Fresh fish. How big, how often? Oh, every day. Her husband keeps fish in the rice field. He brings a fresh one home every day. Continuing interviews revealed the facts. Simina had been married since she was 15; she had borne three children, two of whom had died; and she really didn't have a husband who brought her a fish every day; he had deserted her six months ago! Simina's mother now appeared on the scene. She had come to Simina's house to take care of Simina's small child for the day, but a week of this was too much.

She thought all this fuss and bother with the doctors was a bad joke, and Simina was better off just to return home.

The Cicendo Hospital did not possess an operable fundus camera, so Dr. Sommer packed Simina, her mother, baby, and four interested Cicendo ophthalmologists into a project vehicle for a trip to Jakarta. While there they took colored photographs of Simina's eye lesions and a fluorescence angiography test. Before returning to Bandung they had lunch at a restaurant. After ordering a balanced meal for Simina, they watched in astonishment as she carefully scraped all of the meat and vegetables to the side of her plate and ate only the rice. Simina returned to Cicendo for follow-up examinations. The final analysis, complete with photographs, was embodied in the first paper of the project which was published in the Archives of Ophthalmology, one of the leading ophthalmology publications in the U.S.

Leadership for Studies II and III went to Dr. Sommer by default. For some reason, perhaps their scientific complexity, the Indonesian project leadership just didn't give these studies very great attention. Dr. Sugana provided an ophthalmologist and the hospital space and saw to it that hospital staff cooperated; Tarwotjo found a nutritionist; other staff performed the necessary administrative and statistical tasks; but Indonesian leadership did not translate the manual, give enumerators training in the use of the forms, or pay particular attention to the day-to-day conduct of these studies.

Indonesian Leadership

Study IV was a different matter. Once the site selection was completed, as discussed in Chapter 8, the Indonesian staff assumed entire responsibility for the survey. For Study IV, Dr. Sommer truly served as an advisor, while the Indonesians truly exercised project leadership, making all of the decisions. One may speculate as to the reasons. This was the part of the project which could produce timely data needed for development of the third five-year plan. Possibly it was the part Tarwotjo had chosen to use for his Ph. D. thesis. Most important, though, was the fact that Indonesians had allowed Sommer to take the lead in previous studies. They had benefited from his advice and tutelage. Now they were in a position to prepare and conduct their own survey with minimum help, and they apparently were determined to do just that.

Language and Communications

The vast majority of project employees spoke almost no English. It became obvious that for the simplest communications the Americans would have to use the Indonesian language, Bahasa Indonesia, but it wasn't that easy. From the earliest days of the project, non-English speaking nurses brought children into the office for xerophthalmia examinations. They had to be given some kind of instructions about return visits and the like. While the office secretaries were quite helpful, a call on them each time was an indirect, time-consuming method which interrupted their work.

During the first months of the project, Soemantri, the finance officer, arose early every morning to struggle with his English language tapes. When Fritz, the HKI liaison officer, arrived on the scene, Soemantri proudly told him of his efforts. It shortly became obvious, however, that English was not always a sufficient means of communications between these two individuals. Soemantri thought about all financial and bookkeeping problems in Dutch, the language of his former employers, though his language of conversation were Bahasa Indonesia, Sunda, and to a limited extent, English. And while the English of Tito and Djoko sounded impressive when they spoke it, there were awkward moments when answers were not relevant to the questions asked. There were moments when secretaries misinterpreted typing instructions. There were embarrassing occasions when statistical clerks continued to stand around after receiving instructions. They just hadn't understood the instructions, sometimes because of language difficulties, but perhaps also because of other barriers.

Luckily, Sommer's summer of language instruction in the Netherlands had given him a head start. Throughout his stay in Indonesia, he carried word lists which he studied during his trips, whether by jeep or airplane. He found the language extremely useful in talks with nurses and nutritionists. When perceiving that an English speaking statistical clerk didn't understand his instruction in English, he repeated it in Indonesian. His requests to the finance and supply officers were often in Indonesian, and he interspersed Indonesian with English in his conversations with Djoko and Tito. A little redundancy didn't hurt.

Forms

Fritz was not on the project very long before he recognized that the administrative and financial chores and representing HKI interests did not take up all of his time. With encouragement from Sommer, he began double checking the census and survey forms, later the initial forms received from the Study I clinical team and the first field work of the Study II team. Except for the ophthalmologic and pediatric sections, these forms were printed in Bahasa Indonesia.

Fritz had to start from scratch, but experience elsewhere had led him to negotiate inclusion of a modest sum for language instruction in his HKI contract. It was a good investment. He rapidly learned all of the existing forms, and a lifetime of experience enabled him to quickly spot errors and inconsistencies which he conveyed to the statistical clerks in short notes written in the Indonesian language. After a while the clerks ceased sending Fritz the forms, though occasionally they presented specific problems they encountered.

Fritz's language capability grew and its value increased. Checking the results of the first field examinations by the Study II team, he found several anomalies. The forms were considerably different than the Study I forms because they had been devised to serve different purposes. Obviously, the enumerators did not understand them. Their misunderstandings were compounded by errors and inconsistencies in the Indonesian language on the forms which had not been adequately checked before printing. Fritz prepared a lecture with notes in Bahasa Indonesia which he delivered to the Study II nurses and enumerators. With some faltering he was also able to answer their questions. Accompanying the team on its next field trip, he spot-checked the forms at the examination site. Thereafter, the enumerators, nurses, dietician, statistical clerks, and even the physicians came to Fritz for advice on problems regarding the forms which bothered them.

Subsequently, a check of the second round of Study I forms revealed some translation errors. By this time Fritz could also translate contracts and reports. Deciding to test his developing skill, he composed a much needed Study II field operations manual in Bahasa Indonesia with occasional use of an Indonesian-English dictionary. He reviewed the manual first with his language teacher, then with the statistical staff before he had it typed and distributed. From then on, some project staff refused to let Fritz talk to them in English.

Language Concepts and Cooperation

But language was not the only communications problem; concepts also raised difficulties. Before finalizing the manual for Study II field examinations, the Americans met with the Study II physicians and statistical staff to ensure mutual understanding of remaining problems. One problem raised was the age of children to be examined in the field. It was agreed that all children aged 0-7 would be examined.

Ten days after the manual was distributed, the statistical staff complained that forms of seven-year-old children showed they had not been examined. Another meeting was held. The ophthalmologist explained that she examined all children seven years of age. However, she did not examine children who had already completed seven years, as they were more than seven years old. Since the pattern was now clear, the manual was amended so that all children would be examined between the ages of 0 and 6 years, 11 months and 29 days.

Good communications also require, among other things, a will on the part of everyone in the system to actually communicate. It seemed at times that some Indonesian project members did not always wish to communicate or that they wanted to communicate something special which could only be done in indirect fashion.

Strongly religious members of the general support staff disappeared from the office for an hour or so on Friday at noon to attend mosque services. On one such occasion, a Study II nurse came to Mr. Fritz and asked for alcohol. After checking the storage cabinet to find none there, Fritz awaited the return of the supply officer, who after being informed of the problem went out to purchase the alcohol. The following Friday at noon the nurse came to Fritz with another request. On the third Friday, he noted a Study II nurse making a request of Dr. Sommer. Subsequently Dr. Sommer asked the Study II ophthalmologist why they didn't submit their requests to the supply officer. She replied that he was insufficiently responsive. In fact, Study II was having a very difficult time obtaining vehicles when needed. Looking into this, Dr. Sommer learned that Study II staff were submitting notifications of field visits so late that local authorities sometimes were unprepared to receive the team; thus vehicles had been despatched on useless trips. A subsequent meeting arranged by Dr. Sommer led to resolution of the problem among all parties. The Study II team would present weekly requirements to which the supply officer would respond in timely fashion.

Lebaran is a two-day holiday marking the end of the Muslim fasting month. Because of experiences gained in 1976, the project leadership decided to close down operations for the whole Lebaran week during mid-September 1977. The following week Dr. Sugana decided to make an unannounced field trip to observe Study I operations. The team was nowhere to be found, and Dr. Sugana learned they had decided to take an extra week off in Bali.

The following week the Study I leader was "invited" to a meeting with headquarters personnel. Explaining his action, the Study I chief said he had previously surveyed local authorities and determined that a large percentage of people in the study area would be absent during the week after Lebaran. Project leaders remarked that this was fine, but that good management practices and the responsibility of project headquarters to Jakarta dictated that such matters be communicated beforehand and resolved in consultation with project headquarters. The Study I chief promised that he would do this in the future, but also expressed the hope that future project headquarters' decisions on holidays would be conveyed to him, as he had a responsibility to his team. While the Americans took it for granted that Indonesian project leaders had communicated their decision on holidays to Study I, in fact they had not done so.

In early December 1977, while discussing some technical details with Dr. Sommer, the Study II ophthalmologist casually mentioned that "we've decided" to stop sending Study II patients to the H. S. Hospital for bone marrow biopsies. After Dr. Sommer recovered from this shock, he asked how long this had been going on. Since the beginning of Study II, "somebody" had agreed to send all Study II patients to somebody else's unrelated research study, accompanied by a Study II nurse and conveyed in a project vehicle. No wonder Study II nurses felt overworked; project vehicles were in demand, and the children's parents were reluctant to return with posttreatment patients for follow-up examinations.

Vacations.

A few days later, a Study II physician informed Dr. Sommer that she intended to take a two week vacation beginning on Christmas. Dr. Sommer asked if there were a hospital physician who could replace her. Yes, Dr. "so-and-so" could replace her. If that's so, was Al Sommer's reply, then she should make sure that this physician worked with her in the clinic and the field for a few days before she went on vacation. Dr. Sommer saw both physicians off and on over the next few days, but never saw them together and never saw the replacement physician in the clinic. About December 23, a project secretary asked Fritz if he knew the whole Study II team was planning a vacation. He didn't, though he had wondered at the lack of patients in the ward and that the Study II team was working so hard scrubbing the floors. Sure enough, on the day in question only one nurse showed up. Also, only one patient showed up for a follow-up examination, having been unable to come on the day of appointment. Obviously, the physician had asked hospital authorities not to refer new patients to the Study II Clinic while she and the rest of the team were on vacation.

Training of Personnel

Important elements of many technical assistance activities are the training and further development of host country personnel and the building of institutions. In the case under study, these were not intended to be important elements. The project was intended to be a research activity, not a training activity. Once the activity ended, project personnel would be disbanded, some returning to full-time positions in parent organizations which hopefully would gain from the new knowledge and skills they brought back with them. Others would be unemployed and have to seek other jobs.

Training was an integral part of the project. We have referred to the training of nurses, nutritionists, and enumerators in previous chapters. In a sense, this was more like orientation to the project than real training, although it imparted skills in interviewing and survey techniques, diagnosing eye disease, using laboratory and clinical equipment, and interpreting data.

Nevertheless, research provides excellent training for those who participate in it. It is fair to say that most project personnel had no real appreciation of research before joining the project. But the use of research principles and techniques makes its imprint. All professional employees learned to inquire into aspects of their profession in which they had little previous interest. All employees taxed previous skills to the limit and thereby developed their skills to a higher level.

While not a part of the project proposal, Dr. Sommer imparted a significant amount of training on an informal basis. His work with the hospital physicians, described earlier in this chapter, is an example, although not strictly speaking related to the project. There are other illustrations within the project. For example, when discussing the choice of villages for Study I or the selection of sample sites for Study IV, Dr. Sommer frequently went to the blackboard and lapsed into a professorial mode. As project staff evinced further interest in the principles he set forth, he ordered texts in statistics, sampling, and epidemiology which he encouraged his Indonesian colleagues to study. He also suggested to a number of personnel that they write analytical articles on their work for publication in Indonesian professional journals. During the course of preparing such articles, they came to him for help and suggestions which he provided.

By March 1978 it became obvious that a number of project participants would be responsible for the analysis of data and the publication of research findings; the process had to be systematized. It was agreed that a series of workshops would be held. The first was a general workshop of all senior project personnel and interested parties to review general principles of data analysis, statistical methods, epidemiological principles, approaches to framing questions, ways of designing the analysis to answer these questions, and techniques for reaching the relevant conclusions.

Specific workshops would then be held, attended by headquarters staff and principal members of each study to discuss the questions to be answered by that particular study, to design an analysis of the data to answer those questions, and to assign responsibility for specific data analysis. Statistics personnel would work closely with the responsible individuals. Follow-up workshops would include presentation of analyses and conclusions, at which time questions would be raised, conclusions challenged, and suggestions offered for improvement.

Project planners also agreed to hold an additional general workshop to review principles to prepare manuscripts for publication. Thereafter each person responsible for analyzing data would be expected to prepare a manuscript. Each manuscript would be presented to the group as a whole for criticism and suggestions at follow-up meetings. In addition, the project established a publications committee which would provide written clearances before presentations of talks at professional meetings or submission of articles to journals.

To the extent that project participants continued their enthusiasm for research and writing into their postproject assignments, it was clear that the results of technical assistance would extend beyond the limits of the original research objectives.

10 Synthesizing Preliminary Data

During early January 1978, Dr. Susan Pettiss, Director of Blindness Prevention for HKI in New York, visited Indonesia once again. Project planners were tabulating preliminary data and beginning to think of preliminary steps to recommend in preparation for postresearch action. Dr. Pettiss also needed to confer with her colleagues in Indonesia in connection with HKI's first "annual" report to AID, which according to the contract was due one year after the beginning of Phase II, the operational phase.

Project leaders requested Professor Sulianti Sarosa to convene a steering committee meeting to review preliminary data and propose the next steps. Bandung personnel tried to set the meeting for January 12. Thus, Dr. Pettiss could attend the meeting and meet with other agencies in Jakarta, such as USAID, UNICEF, and the Lions Club, prior to departure for Bangladesh on January 16.

On January 6, Tarwotjo received a call from Dr. Sulianti's office in Jakarta. The steering committee meeting would be held at her house the following morning at 10:30. The next morning, Saturday, Pettiss, Sommer, and Fritz left Bandung by car at 5:30. Traffic was light, the sky was unusually clear, and they enjoyed marvelous and spectacular scenery during their uniquely speedy three and a half hour journey to Jakarta. At the Nutrition Academy, they met Tarwotjo, Djoko, and Muhilal. The latter two had just arrived from Bogor. Tarwotjo had difficulties contacting other committee members, and no others were present. They reviewed the program they wished to present, and at 10:30 appeared at the front door of Professor Sulianti Sarosa's house.

Professor Sulianti Sarosa was meeting with someone else. Inviting the group inside, she exclaimed that she hadn't expected so many. She had requested that anyone coming from Bandung that weekend should bring for her signature the invitational letter for next Thursday's steering committee meeting, but no one had brought the invitation. That afternoon Pettiss, Sommer, and Fritz drove back through crowded weekend traffic, mist, and heavy rain to Bandung.

The meeting held the following Wednesday was successful. At a time when the project was halfway through its operational stage, the Indonesians reconfirmed their vital stake in the project. They presented the data, they reviewed the findings, and they reviewed the next steps to be taken within the framework of Indonesian national mechanisms.

FINDINGS: STUDY I

The Study I team had almost completed its third clinical round of preschool children in the Purwakarta area. The prevalence of clinical xerophthalmia was substantial, averaging 7.4% on the first round. The rate of active corneal involvement was also high, four cases among 3,800 children or ten times the WHO criterion for a significant public health problem. Half of the active noncorneal cases underwent spontaneous remission or "self-cure" during the three and a half months between the first and second clinical rounds. However, the incidence of new cases in the same interval was 2.6%. Serum vitamin A levels were highly correlated with abnormal cases. Levels among sufferers of night blindness were almost as low as those with conjunctival xerosis.

Initially, Dr. Sommer had been somewhat reluctant to include night blindness in the Study I examinations because it would be difficult to determine if the children were night blind or not. The Study I ophthalmologist had an interest in the subject, however, and Dr. Sommer encouraged him to go ahead. Night blindness was a common complaint in the Sunda area, and the Sundanese had a term for it in their language. By asking the right questions Dr. Hussaini found he could get correct answers from the child's mother. Later, on a sample basis, he visited homes of night blind children during the evening and tested their ability to find familiar objects placed close to them. When the blood results came in, they correlated more closely with the mothers' histories than with the clinical tests. Investigators remained reluctant to recommend Dr. Hussaini's questions to clinicians in other countries, however, believing they were culture specific and not transferable without adaptation, trial, and error.

Serum vitamin A levels among matched controls were midway between those of abnormals and random samples, suggesting that vitamin A deficiency was a community or locale-specific problem. Carotene levels followed the same pattern as vitamin A levels, apparently confirming that children with better vitamin A levels consumed more food containing carotene. This very useful biochemical check provided the basis for one of the few validations of dietary data ever to be published.

STUDY II AND III FINDINGS

Studies II and III had investigated 82 children with active corneal disease and an additional 66 children with night blindness or Bitot's Spots with conjunctival xerosis. Vitamin A was the principal etiology in all xerophthalmia cases, but one third of the cases with classical corneal xerosis were otherwise healthy and well-nourished. Thus protein energy malnutrition was not a requirement, as previously thought. On the other hand, investigations indicated that keratomalacia almost certainly involved defects in protein metabolism. Whether vitamin A deficiency was similarly important was not yet clear. The number of cases to date, however, was inadequate for definite conclusions.

STUDY IV FINDINGS

Having completed their sample surveys in Bali, Lombok, and Java, the three Study IV teams were now on Sumatra and Ambon. They had found a prevalence of active corneal cases far exceeding WHO criteria for a "significant problem" in all the provinces to date. However, they had detected only negligible numbers of corneal scars, suggesting mortality in an extraordinary number of cases. This appeared significant, as prior assumptions were that only 50% of such children died.

Dietary data suggested that vitamin A fortification of wheat flour, monosodiumglutamate, or refined sugar might result in a significant reduction in the incidence of xerophthalmia. For example, 73% of the cases in Central Java reportedly ingested a minimum of 15 grams of wheat per month. Government policy had already been formulated for the fortification of wheat flour, but no determination had been made of the kinds and quantities of fortification materials to be used.

Government officers were careful not to proceed with the premature action. They recommended a series of technical seminars to discuss the findings with others experienced in vitamin A matters and to review the matter of fortification with an interministerial committee already set up for the purpose. After that, feasibility and impact studies would be carried out.

Data Compilation: Problems

It will be recalled that the project had contracted with the computer center at the Institute of Technology (ITB) in Bandung for its card punching and computer programming. ITB had assigned a young programmer, Urip, to work on the project. After some false starts, it developed that he was not available full time; his principal job was in Jakarta, and he was in Bandung only two days a week. Nevertheless, he was quite helpful in preparing initial programs which assisted the statistical group in ironing out some data problems.

After the steering committee meeting in January 1978, Al Sommer developed a manual of initial programs which he reviewed with headquarter's staff. He then asked that a meeting be set up with ITB. No one at ITB was available for two weeks. Moreover, Urip was in Jakarta preparing for a trip to Paris. In fact, he had been awarded a French government study grant and would be gone for three to five years. After the steering committee meeting was over and Dr. Pettiss had departed, Sommer and Fritz sat down at their separate desks and began to review the facts at hand. This was particularly important for Dr. Sommer because he had to prepare for a February meeting of the HKI Advisory Committee on Blindness Prevention in New York.

DATA INTERPRETATION

There was no doubt that nutritional blindness, or xerophthalmia was a significant problem in Indonesia. During a six-month period, 190 cases of corneal involvement had appeared at the Cicendo Eye Hospital and the Cikampek Clinic. Moreover, compilation of data secured from the first two rounds of Study I examinations had resulted in the first annual incidence rates, four per thousand for corneal disease and 104 per thousand for noncorneal disease. Study IV data already obtained for a sampling of the vast majority of the Indonesian population which lived in Java and Bali (according to the Statistical Yearbook of Indonesia of 1975, more than 88 million of Indonesia's population of 118 million lived in Java and Bali) confirmed the widespread prevalence of xerophthalmia.

Dr. Sommer made a few calculations. Estimating a population of 12 million Indonesian children aged one-five, the years of greatest risk, an annual incidence of 4:1,000 would result in 48,000 corneal cases per year and an incidence of 104:1,000 would mean an astounding one and a quarter million noncorneal cases per year.

From the outset, it was anticipated that research would confirm xerophthalmia as a major cause of blindness in Indonesia. Other findings were more disturbing. The Study IV countrywide survey had produced prevalence rates for active corneal diseases of nearly 1:1,000. However, the scar rate was only one fifth of that and as a cumulative phenomenon, there should have been 25 times as many scars as those found. The only explanation was that over 90% of blinded children must be dying. Xerophthalmia had a high mortality rate and was directly responsible for a large proportion of Indonesia's childhood mortality.

In considering the Indonesian mortality rate, there was no doubt that malnutrition and systemic diseases accounted for many deaths, but for many others, there appeared to be only one explanation. A large proportion seemed to be dying because poor families, where mothers had many conflicting economic and home care responsibilities, could not give these helpless children the care they needed.

PROPOSED THERAPY

From Study II data noted in connection with the steering committee meeting, it was clear that vitamin A deficiency was responsible for nutritional eye disease in the vast majority of cases, but it was necessary to determine the most practical form of vitamin A therapy. Until then the general recommendations called for intramuscular administration of 100,000 IU (international units) water miscible vitamin A upon diagnosis, with an additional oral dose the following day. But intramuscular vitamin A was impractical for most rural Indonesian dispensaries; it was too expensive, had a short shelf life, and required needles, syringes, and strict sterile techniques. Oral, oil miscible vitamin A suffered none of these shortcomings. Moreover, preliminary Study II results indicated oral administration of 200,000 IU oil miscible vitamin A on two successive days was as clinically effective as previously recommended treatment. Single doses of either intramuscular or oral vitamin A had proven inadequate for severely malnourished children, many of whom relapsed in one month.

What was the best method for increasing vitamin A intake to prevent eye disease? The most rapidly effective means was artificial provision of supplemental vitamin A. A potentially long-term solution was to promote natural dietary sources of vitamin A and provitamin A carotenoids. Such promotion would have to be undertaken through health education activities. Data from Studies I and IV already confirmed that xerophthalmia children were found largely in backward, traditional areas. Educational influences would tend to spread slowly in such environments.

Though supplemental vitamin A capsules were inexpensive, their mass distribution had proven expensive and logistically difficult within the Indonesian system. Actual acceptance was uncertain, and the drop-out rate was high. However, it might be the only feasible approach for some areas in the immediate future. The possibility of food fortification appeared to offer fairly immediate opportunities. It could be rapidly effective, and the use of regular marketing channels minimized distribution costs. The major challenge was to identify the most suitable food product for fortification. It must be a product eaten generally by children susceptible to xerophthalmia. Amounts consumed would have to fall within a particular range to avoid provision of too much vitamin A to persons eating large quantities of the product. The product would also have to be centrally processed in a minimum number of locations in order to minimize problems of administration, logistics, and control.

Dr. Sommer put the above thoughts, along with some recommendations, into a paper which he called "Major Topics for Review," expecting to present it to the HKI Advisory Committee at its New York meeting on February 25. Meanwhile, Fritz was also cogitating. He had earlier requested AID in Washington for information which might be useful in carrying out feasibility studies of possible fortification programs. A number of books on the subject had now arrived, and he studied them assiduously and took notes. He put his thoughts into a paper which he called "A Discussion of Possible Vitamin A Intervention Programs in Indonesia." He covered nutritional education, changes in food production, supplementary feeding programs, public health activities, new food products like weaning foods, enrichment or fortification of existing foods, and periodic massive doses of vitamin A.

Fritz touched on all of these possible intervention programs, coming to conclusions similar to those of Dr. Sommer. Both started from the premise that the primary target of intervention programs was rural, pre-school children and that the programs should be of least cost with most speedy possible coverage of the target population on a permanent basis. With regard to agricultural efforts, Fritz noted an Indian study which indicated that meeting vitamin and mineral deficiencies through fruit and vegetable production was 70-1,000 times more expensive than synthetically produced ingredients. (1) Another study indicated that preformed vitamin A is four to six times as efficient as beta carotene because much of the latter is lost during the process of absorption and conversion before it can be utilized by the human organism. (2)

Of course, no one intervention would solve the problem. Probably a combination of interventions would be required which would address short-term, intermediate, and long-term solutions. However, as recognized elsewhere, "Modification of patterns pertaining to production and consumption through socioeconomic, agricultural, and educational measures which would be the permanent solution to the vitamin A deficiency problem would take a long time. However, the extent of the problem is such that application of more rapid emergency measures is justified." (3)

Study IV data had shown that the majority of children with xerophthalmia in Bali and Java consumed wheat flour, monosodiumglutamate (MSG), sugar, and candies (see Table 10.1). One would not attempt to fortify candy directly, because it was manufactured in many locations. If sugar were fortified, it could be used in the candy.

Table 10.1. Percentage of Xerophthalmia Children Who Consume Potentially Fortifiable Foods at Least Once Weekly: Preliminary Study IV Results

	Wheat	Sugar	MSG	Candies
Lombok	47.1	56.6	37.6	37.8
Bali	66.7	74.1	77.8	44.4
East Java	52.8	66.0	77.4	49.0
Central Java	47.2	62.8	87.1	47.0
West Java	44.3	23.7	81.4	67.1

Fortification of these products had already been practiced in other developing countries. Vitamin A had been added to MSG for a three province pilot project in the Philippines and to sugar in Central America. Wheat in India had been fortified with a number of ingredients, including vitamin A. Moreover, the Massachusetts Institute of Technology (MIT) had already prepared a report for WHO which strongly recommended the fortification of wheat flour in Indonesia with a number of ingredients, including vitamin A. (4)

All the studies Fritz read indicated that fortification represented a minor portion of production costs. MIT had estimated, for example, a 1% increase in the cost of wheat flour after fortification with thiamine, riboflavin, niacin, iron, calcium, and vitamin A.

Precautions in Food Fortification

Whatever product was fortified, some people would eat it who were not susceptible to xerophthalmia, some every day. Care would have to be exercised to assure that such individuals did not receive too much vitamin A. On the other hand, some persons at risk would eat the product rarely, or in the case of wheat flour, in a mixture with unfortified products like cassava flour. Thus some children would not get adequate vitamin A through fortification alone. So there probably was a need for periodic distribution of the massive dose capsule in particular areas like Lombok and Northern Sumatra, where Study IV data showed that a large proportion of the children consumed little or none of the fortifiable products. There were many other areas where the community health center could retain capsule supplies for preventing and controlling xerophthalmia. Since no single suggested fortifiable product would reach all children at risk, the project still needed to analyze whether a combination of fortified products would raise the percentage significantly and whether this could be done.

Wheat was an important product. Its use was increasing as shown by import statistics. The wheat was processed into flour in three mills in Indonesia, thus making administration, logistics, and control practical. MIT had reported that some of the mills already possessed the necessary equipment, and it recommended a "standard wheat enrichment formula" which could be purchased from a reputable international firm as a premix.

Fritz decided to discuss MSG possibilities with Al Sommer. Was it not possible to cut costs and aim more sharply at the target group by setting up two processing lines at the MSG plant, fortifying the material in one line which fed into a family size packet, while leaving unfortified the other line feeding into an institutional size container? Al agreed this seemed a practical idea.

And while considering the targeting of specific classes of consumers, what about wheat flour? The MIT report had concluded that wheat flour was consumed "primarily in urban and primarily by middle- and upper-income groups." (5) Study IV data obtained so far, however, indicated that both xerophthalmia children and a broad random sample of children consumed wheat flour products. Could it be that poor people were getting a different grade of flour than the higher income groups? Tarwotjo promised to look into the matter.

Sugar also seemed a practical vehicle for fortification. The process of vitamin A fortification was known because the project possessed a rather complete technical description of the Central American sugar fortification process, including analyses of the various decisions that had to be made. (6) Costs were low but the number of sugar refineries that produced sugar in Indonesia seemed to be in dispute. More accurate information was needed.

Recommendations

Fritz ended his paper with recommendations for (a) a working committee to review existing data, seek additional data, and design feasibility studies to recommend to the government's technical committee, (b) the early involvement of concerned international agencies, (c) participation by commercial and other food technology and nutrition experts, and (d) sending Indonesian experts for short trips abroad to observe firsthand the fortification experiences of other countries. He also mentioned a number of other steps to be taken, e. g., market analysis; stability, settling, taste, and acceptability trials; decisions on equipment; cost analysis; and the preparation of mandatory fortification statutes to be passed by the government. Dr. Sommer took copies of this paper as well as his own to present to the advisory committee in New York, but first Al had to attend a WHO meeting in Geneva. While there, his wife called from Bandung. An emergency medical problem required the attention of a physician in Singapore. Before leaving Geneva for the return to Indonesia, Al discussed the papers with Susan Pettiss who also had been attending the WHO meeting. She would present Al's report at the advisory committee meeting on February 25.

Meanwhile, on February 15, a number of project participants and associates attended a vitamin A seminar at Bogor. Dr. Glover presented a learned lecture on the biochemistry of vitamin A in the human body. Sandy Hui, a Hong Kong representative of Hoffman La Roche, an international firm which had pioneered in vitamin A technology, presented a lecture on that topic. The meeting provided an opportunity for an exchange of ideas, opinions, facts, questions, and answers.

Tarwotjo had been talking to the Industry Department and confirmed that high grade wheat flour tended to go to bakers of bread consumed by higher income levels, while lower grades tended to be used in products more commonly eaten by poorer people. This offered a real opportunity to target the fortified product for the population most in need of vitamin A and to avoid the risk of toxicity for maximum consumers. Sandy Hui confirmed Fritz's notion about the possibility of segregating fortified MSG for family consumption. He announced that the vitamin A program just launched in the Philippines was doing exactly that.

There was some discussion about the possibility of fortifying salt. Most project planners had been dubious about the suitability of salt as a vehicle for vitamin A fortification. It was produced in many different places under conditions which presented obstacles to standardization. One participant in the meeting, however, advocated salt, saying the government had decided to standardize salt and to purchase all "people-produced" salt. Someone else spoke up to say that while this was true, in actual practice it would be a long time before salt could satisfy the vitamin A fortification criterion on a national basis. Naturally, the ideas were not final, but they provided a basis for further study which hopefully would lead to meaningful action.

COMPUTER REQUIREMENTS

After Urip left for Paris, Al Sommer conversed further with ITB representatives to see what should be done next about computer requirements. Who would do our programming now? Well, sad to say, ITB didn't have anyone else right now, but perhaps next May one or two programmers "might" return from training in Paris. Al wasn't satisfied with this. He and Tarwotjo began talking to a firm in Jakarta. One bright programmer seemed quite interested and spent several hours discussing the project and its analytical requirements with Al Sommer in his Jakarta hotel room. Al drew up some requirements, the Jakarta firm provided some estimates, and project heads were convinced that computer requirements were soon to be satisfied.

It was difficult to get all parties together for a meeting. However, on June 12, 1978 three representatives of the Jakarta firm came to Bandung by early morning train. They had questions to sort out, many of which could best be answered by Djoko who was still in Bogor because his wife had just delivered their third little daughter.

During the sessions Al asked the programmer if he could stay overnight. It was obvious their business could not be concluded in one day. The programmer replied that he had hoped the business could be concluded in one day because he would be tied up in Jakarta for the rest of the week. Al asked, "Well, how about coming back again next Monday? Then we can settle the remaining questions with Djoko," but the programmer replied, "Oh, I'm sorry, but I can't. I'm going on two weeks vacation." When Al responded, "Well, we've waited long enough already. We can wait for a couple more weeks. When can you come?" The programmer answered, "Oh, I'm afraid I cannot come back again. You see, I am leaving the firm." Al remained depressed for two or three days after that.

After discussions with a senior officer of the firm, however, project officers decided to keep trying. During the last week of June, two programmers arrived in Bandung. As conversations proceeded, they and Djoko went to ITB for discussions. While there they looked into the organization of the punch cards. What they found was a bit distressing.

Only a portion of the cards punched had the necessary printed information on them. To review these and correct the omissions would require a month. In addition, cards punched for Studies I and IV had been stored together. Worse, however, was trying to locate cards punched for the Study I census survey; project officers were told that Urip had taken them to Jakarta, but he was now in Paris, and no one knew where he left the cards.

UNFORESEEN PROBLEMS

> ...each project comes into the world accompanied by two sets of partially or wholly offsetting potential developments: (1) a set of possible and unsuspected threats to its profitability and existence and (2) a set of unsuspected remedial actions that can be taken should a threat become real...(7)

Inaccurate Accusations

In late May 1978 a second AID evaluation team visited the project. Before beginning one of the meetings with project staff, one of the evaluators opened a typed letter which had been handed to him at his hotel. The letter seemed peculiar, having been typed on two typewriters. Though unsigned, the name appearing at the bottom belonged to one of the young statistical clerks hired to work on Study II data until the end of June. The letter complained that the project was claiming normal children as abnormal and appended some tables with names of children, diagnosis classification, and serum vitamin A blood values. The writer went on to say that he was submitting this data to prevent waste of United States government money. Djoko confronted his clerk with the letter. The clerk became very angry and swore he had nothing to do with the letter.

After the evaluation team left Indonesia, Tarwotjo and Tito discussed the matter with Retno and Apong, another statistical clerk and the chief nurse of Study II, respectively. These women obtained their original data on the children in question and compared them with data presented with the letter. They found blood values submitted with the letter were not based on the affected children's initial examination. For the most part they were based on posttreatment blood samples. In some cases they turned out to belong to the affected child's matched control, a normal child of the same age and sex. Who had written the letter? As the four project officers examined the various documents involved, one of the firls remarked that she had never previously seen the particular form attached to the letter. It so happened that Isnodi, the supply officer, kept copies of all forms printed by the project, along with names of persons ordering them. His records showed that the original suspect had requested the printing of this form.

In two hours of quiet Javanese conversation, Tarwotjo secured a confession from the culprit. He apparently hadn't realized his data were false. Apparently his motives were sincere. Why he presented the false data to a visiting team instead of asking advice from his supervisor was not clarified. Moreover, he was not fired, and he stayed on the job until the end of June, his originally scheduled date of departure from the project.

11 Conclusions: Agenda for the Future

LESSONS LEARNED

> ...systematic attention needs be paid not only to the various aspects of implementation at the level of a project but also to factors which are beyond the control of the project's management. (1)

As this final chapter was being written, the project, though on target, was far from completion. None of the four major studies had been finished. The bulk of the analytical work still had to be done. Many problems lay ahead. But the main outlines of research results were already clearly seen - and for the purpose of this Case Study in technical assistance (TA), it is hoped that some lessons had already been learned.

The first and most obvious lesson is that unpredictable events sometimes occur in a comprehensive TA project.

1. Government agreement was delayed.

2. Budgets had to be reinterpreted.

3. Available personnel turned out to be unavailable.

4. Research subjects became uncooperative.

5. Equipment did not arrive on time, and sometimes did not work properly after arrival.

6. People had accidents, others got sick, and babies were born. One key professional died.

7. Transportation and communications were imperfect.

Project leaders had continued cause to wonder whether their plans had been somewhat short of perfect. Their most chronic problems, computer programming and biochemistry, led them to wonder whether their plans should have included a full-time programmer and biochemist complete with lab rather than to attempt to rely as they had completely on associates outside the formal organization of the project for these services.

Lesson One: Murphy's Law

If they had it to do over, perhaps they would do things differently. On the other hand, this wouldn't guarantee problem-free results. It was best that they learn to live by what Al Sommer continually referred to as Murphy's Law, "If there's a chance that something will go wrong, it will."

Lesson Two: Participants' Initiative

The second lesson was that given adequate skills, experience, and initiative on the part of project participants, sufficient delegation of authority to them, and perhaps a bit of help when needed and requested, people on the scene could work with these unpredictable problems and solve most of them, as they had:

1. Project participants doubled their efforts to assure that the project remained on schedule.

2. Project participants learned to compromise with budgets and to arrange tradeoffs.

3. Project participants found alternative personnel or alternate methods of getting things done.

4. A part-time associate of the project, a social worker, intervened to influence a change in research subjects' attitudes.

5. HKI purchased locally available equipment, and USAID in Jakarta arranged finances for rental of vehicles.

6. Not all problems were solved.

Lesson Three: Sponsoring Agencies' Flexibility

For many discerning individuals, these two lessons, once learned, will lead logically to the third lesson: that agencies sponsoring and financing international TA efforts should not insist that implementing agencies adhere to every detail of initial project plans because those plans inevitably will be modified, as this project had experienced:

1. A Study I team headquarters was established and an extra vehicle employed for the reasons described in Chapter 4.

2. The nature of Study III was drastically revised for reasons described in Chapter 5.

3. Drawing of blood had to be drastically reduced because of problems described in Chapters 5 and 6.

4. Unforeseen purchases of equipment were made for reasons described in Chapters 5 and 6.

5. Assistance from USAID in Jakarta was secured for renting vehicles at the beginning of Study IV because of late delivery of American jeeps as described in Chapters 6, 7, and 8.

Lesson Four: Flexibility of Plans

To predict that plans will need to change is tantamount to the judgment that project plans and contracts should contain an element of flexibility which permits such change, which is lesson four.

The author suggests that good technical assistance planning is more than preparation of personnel lists, organization charts, bills of materials, budgets, and schedules of actions and critical events. A planner hopefully wants to accomplish more than completion of a plan. He is planning for sound implementation of a project which requires some additional perspective, the perspective of future unpredictable contingencies. Despite the unpredictable nature of particular contingencies, however, we have ample experience to demonstrate that contingencies will occur, no matter how perfect the plan. This calls for a degree of flexibility in the plan and recognition that it is a continuous process, requiring adaptation, modification, and overhaul during the course of implementation.

Plans: Inflexibility and Possible Consequences

Unfortunately, the author has encountered some people engaged in technical assistance policy and procedures planning, financing, and contracting who believe that adjustments in plans are disguised attempts to hoodwink the financial sponsor. To them, the burden of proof is on the implementing agent, and they feel compelled to structure the contractual fine print to guarantee that the implementing agent is held responsible.

One favorite restriction is to require the contractor to obtain consent from the AID's contracting officer in advance of any "major change" in project plans. One can readily imagine the confusion and delays which such restrictions might have caused under the circumstances described in this case study. First, who would determine that changed plans were in fact "major?" A squeamish TA team leader would have considered any change as falling in that category, whereas a bold leader would have considered all changes as being minor. Second, though the HKI contract was with AID in Washington, the mission director (USAID in Jakarta), was "the chief representative of AID in the Cooperating Country." The fine print of the HKI contract says that "Although the Contractor will be responsible for all professional and technical details of the work called for by the contract, he shall be under the general policy guidance of the Mission Director and shall keep the Mission Director currently informed of the progress of the work under the contract." The TA team leader certainly would be wary of informing the mission director about proposed changes in plans before proposing them to HKI in New York. Such action might lead to knowledge of the proposal by AID in Washington before HKI headquarters had decided what to do, i.e., whether to get the contracting officer's approval or to suggest an alternative. When the contracting officer finally received the proposal, he would want to refer it to the responsible technical officer, who would want to refer it to his boss, who would want to hold a meeting on the subject. And just to carry the matter a bit further, suppose the Indonesians did not agree with the final decisions?

The Indonesian Project: Flexibility and Success

Luckily, few restrictions imposed upon this project were of an onerous nature. In fact, the contract contained an element of budgetary flexibility for which project implementers were exceedingly grateful. The contractor was allowed to "exceed the dollar costs of any individual line item as reasonably necessary for completion of the research effort." The total budget was a restriction, of course, as were rules for payment of salaries and allowances, but these were reasonable and could be followed.

Project objectives are the important thing. The HKI contract spelled these out, provided an outline of the studies required to achieve those objectives, and incorporated the contractor's unsolicited proposal. The proposal itself listed certain foreseen problems. While it was quite a comprehensive proposal, it did not, on the whole, pin down the exact methodology for carrying out each study. After all, it was a research project, and research requires an experimental approach. If one line of action does not produce a valid response, then the investigator backs up and plans an alternate line of action.

The project was not a highly structured activity. It stuck to its main goals, and project leaders shifted attention and personnel resources from one to another as needed. They avoided setting up tight organizational compartments which would have led to unbalanced workloads. Though highly directed toward its goals, the project purposefully avoided institutionalization. By June 1978 the Study II and IV teams could disband, and by the end of the year the Study I team would cease operations. Though complete analyses of all data might require some years, project headquarters would fold up by mid-1979. Dr. Sommer would move to New York or London to work on continued analyses. Tarwotjo and Tito would return to Jakarta and Djoko to Bogor. There were some rumors to the effect that Fritz might be required to stay on in Jakarta to work with Tarwotjo and others on continued data analyses and the development of intervention programs, but the project organization was free to disband.

Departure from the original plan

The project departed from original plans in only four <u>major</u> respects. Project planners in Bandung went ahead with these changes because it made sense to do so, and HKI in NY, the AID site visit team, and AID in Washington supported these decisions.

Despite the budgetary flexibility referred to earlier, HKI had difficulties in justifying expenditure overruns on specific line items even though they did not exceed the total budget. For example, up to mid-1978, AID officers in Washington had refused to honor HKI claims for reimbursing the international travel and transportation of the author, his wife, and household effects. The contract had omitted budgetary provision for this item because HKI originally hired a local American to fill the liaison officer position. When this arrangement collapsed, HKI recruited in the United States "as reasonably necessary for completion of the research effort." However, contractual flexibility does not always lead to flexible attitudes by those who review the contractor's claims for reimbursement.

Not only are such bureaucratic attitudes unfortunate in themselves, they sometimes also create unfortunate squeamishness in contractors' attitudes. For instance, possession of Indonesian language ability by the original liaison officer led HKI to limit its budget for language training, but the stateside recruited replacement liaison officer succeeded in bargaining for language training in his employment contract. He started out spending $15 a week for this purpose, then lowered his expenditures to $10. After nearly a year of this, HKI asked him to stop language training because the budgetary item had been exceeded. The liaison officer continued his lessons at his own expense, not only "as reasonably necessary for completion of the research effort," but also for his own personal satisfaction in improving his capability to communicate with Indonesian people on and off the job.

Lesson Five: Delegation of Authority to Representatives

If this case study demonstrates the widely held view of students and practitioners of technical assistance that unpredictable events are inevitable, that problems are best solved by people closest to the scene of action, that the financing agent should not insist on blind adherence to details of initial plans, and that planning in fact should include a degree of flexibility and opportunity for continuous adaptation, then we should derive a fifth lesson: that donor agency headquarters in Washington, New York, Rome, and Geneva in most instances cannot deal adequately with single project emergencies scattered around the globe and hence should delegate maximum authority for dealing with those problems to representatives closest to the scene of action.

During the author's long experience with United States foreign agencies, there have been repeated attempts by Washington officers to decrease delegation of authority to overseas personnel and to hamstring the freedom of TA practitioners. Luckily the project reviewed in this case study did not suffer in this regard. Project participants assumed authority, and they sought help when needed from the nearest capable sources. Given the various relationships which existed among various donor and Indonesian government agencies, it will readily be seen that any real delays or deficiencies in project operations would have been a disaster from which the project could not have recovered.

The first five lessons had to do with TA planning and organization on the donor side. Remaining lessons have to do with TA attitudes and relationships with the recipient government.

Lesson Six: Recipient Governments' Participation

It possibly seems too obvious to say that lesson six is that recipient governments must participate in project planning, but the author has seen many project proposals unilaterally drafted by Americans. He has also seen some proposals which were never implemented, and he has seen some fail during implementation because the host government -- and donor agencies are better prepared if they consider the government as a "host" rather than a "recipient" -- was not deeply committed to the project. It is advantageous if the host government conceives of the problem first and asks for help. Luckily the project under review falls in this category.

Lesson Seven: Recipient Understanding

A seventh lesson is that in activities where the support or participation of many elements of the host government is required, every effort should be made to assure that all elements understand the purposes of the project and their role in it. This is particularly important in village government, but every stage in between may play an unsuspected role, be jealous of its prerogatives, and resentful of unintended neglect.

Lesson Eight: Language and Communication

This leads us to the eighth lesson, the importance of language and effective communication to international TA endeavors. Their importance is frequently underestimated. Officials of TA organizations frequently overestimate the English capability of local project executives. Often, however, even where the local person has enjoyed a modern education and even though he impresses one with his ability to "think" in English, this capability is sometimes a thin veneer covering thick underlying layers of modes of thought, attitudes, societal customs, and beliefs which developed during childhood, within his family, and in the care of a village nursemaid. And his traditions are important to him. A TA expert who attempts to get by without trying to understand the local culture will have difficulty communicating, but he will have some difficulty in any case.

Lesson Nine: American Impatience

Part of the TA specialist's problems, as described heretofore, are what he considers to be the insufficient administrative systems he faces in the foreign assignment. But to be successful in his prime job, lesson nine is it is best that he learn to deal with local administrative systems without expressing too often or too loud his American impatience. In this regard it may be useful to quote from John Montgomery. (2)

> American values such as efficiency, responsibility, and professionalism have dominated all efforts to improve foreign aid procedures, although they are values which are at times irrelevant or even run counter to those of most traditional societies. "Efficiency," a Western and especially American value, calls for the abandonment of many taboos and social traditions, including forms of favoritism that are essential to the family and elite systems of most of the underdeveloped world; "responsibility" implies a delegation of authority and specialization of function that are impossible in much of the world; "professionalism" requires forms of training, the development of a career service, and the introduction of standards that few nonindustrial societies can support.

One must concede that real development and the raising of levels of life of Indonesia's common people requires a relaxation of its rigid administrative procedures. The author's basic training in economics forces him to conclude that a nation's citizens can only share the income it produces. The author's personal observations lead him to believe that millions of manhours are spent annually by government functionaries and their citizen clients in the production of paper work, which produces no income and the purpose of which is often difficult to discern. Some improvements have been made, and hopefully these improvements will spread rapidly.

Lesson Ten: Procurement and Delivery of American Commodities

On the other hand, the tenth lesson is that representatives of the United States find it very difficult to demonstrate the efficiency of American administrative systems and their applicability to local conditions in the face of demonstrated inefficiency in American procurement and delivery of project commodities. One of the problems, from the author's point of view, is that most AID employees no longer feel concerned by delays; over the years they have learned to accept them as a fact of life. When Susan Pettiss of HKI in New York approached AID in Washington with a list of procurement delays, she was unable to locate anyone to admit responsibility for the procurement. In the interest of overall administrative efficiency, AID had centralized its contracting procurement services and organizationally removed them from the geographic country desks, the very units from which such services were most likely to obtain relevant feedback. No one will quarrel with the principle of efficiency if he can locate the responsibility. When he cannot, he begins to wonder.

AID EXPERIENCE: REFLECTIONS

It is difficult for the author to feel dispassionate about AID. He spent 25 years of his life as an employee of the organization in its various forms and under its various names. In earlier years some noted scholars published studies on foreign aid agencies and programs. (3) My findings, which are based solely on experience, are in many ways very similar to theirs.

History of Foreign Aid Programs

Foreign aid is an integral part of American foreign policy. Every United States president since Harry S. Truman has found it essential. Its central theme has been a reflection of United States democratic philosophy and of policy espoused openly by every president since Franklin D. Roosevelt: the improvement of opportunity for the less fortunate members of society and a commitment to the elimination of social injustices and economic inequities.

When dedicated people are assigned important tasks consistent with these aims, they are eager to perform with a high degree of responsibility. The amount of remuneration and position in the organizational heirarchy are less essential than the feeling of self-importance and satisfaction attached to successful performance. But what we see too frequently in AID today are meritorious economic and social programs being carried forward with stilted, brutalizing ridigity by bureaucrats exercising routine procedures. Apparently the visionary zealots of yesteryear have become the hardened, perhaps realistic, bureaucrats of the current AID scene.

What has happened? First, with the possible exception of Point Four, which was administered by the Technical Cooperation Administration during the early 1950s, the central theme of foreign aid, as enunciated by various American administrations, has never been as clear as the statement set forth by the author in the foregoing paragraphs. Rather than function as an instrument of long-range policy for improving international welfare, the program has become a tool for all kinds of short-term, sometimes short-sighted, objectives. Second, because it was easy to debate ad nauseam the various short-term objectives each administration and the Congress imposed on the program, it became a political football in the hands of each incoming administration and for all political shades represented in the United States Congress. To protect itself against continuous and growing Congressional dissatisfaction, each incumbent administration undertook new mammoth studies of the foreign aid agency, usually accompanying each study with disparagement of past programs and the people who ran them and with glowing promises of the far-reaching program achievements and administrative efficiency to result from the latest study. Each reorganization shook up past organizational relationships, leading to "serious delays in both programming and implementation, a lowering of employee morale, and a loss of confidence in the public eye." (4) The personnel turnover resulting from the political nature of the program and general personnel dissatisfaction led to greater knowledge by some Congressmen than those neophyte administration spokesmen who testified on Capitol Hill each succeeding year.

Illustrations

Only a few illustrations are needed to tell the story. After the author began employment with the Economic Cooperation Administration (ECA, Marshall Plan) in 1951, Congress passed legislation which abolished ECA and created the Mutual Security Agency (MSA). About the same time, the president decided that the new aid programs to India and Pakistan should be channeled through the Technical Cooperation Administration (TCA) (Point four) rather than the new MSA. When Fritz sought to make the switch to TCA, he was impolitely challenged by a TCA personnel officer who finally agreed to accept his application for possible future reference. Meanwhile, in accordance with the president's decision, TCA quickly set up an office to plan and conduct programs in India and Pakistan. The people put in charge of the office busily began a search for qualified personnel. Perhaps accidentally, they located the author, a very junior officer with some knowledge of India, a bit of newly gained knowledge about planning foreign aid programs, and a great deal of enthusiasm.

Reporting for work in a temporary World War I building prior to his swearing in, the author was amazed at the high degree of responsibility exercised competently by lower grade officers, some of clerical grade, stationed on the India and Pakistan desks. Upon arrival in India, the author was given responsibility for drafting the basic agreement signed on January 5, 1952 by Prime Minister Jawaharlal Nehru and United States Ambassador Chester Bowles. At a later date, recognizing problems which had arisen in intergovernmental communications and procedures related to program negotiations, Fritz reported these to his director who assigned him the job of working out new procedures with the government of India. His handling of the job led to his assuming responsibility for all negotiations and implementation of technician recruitment and contracting. He was given discretionary authority for the sending of cables to Washington and for communications with contracting agencies. When he handed over his responsibilities to a more senior, professional, personnel officer in 1954, he did so with considerable pride in a job well done. Other junior colleagues of the author also performed high quality, responsible tasks in the early India Point four context.

Stassenization

But the elections of 1952 brought a new administration to power. TCA was merged with the Foreign Operations Administration which had emerged from the Mutual Security Agency. Headed by Harold Stassen, a process was set in motion which was unpopularly referred to as "Stassenization." Stassenization was a reduction in force which drove highly competent foreign aid administrators to the Ford Foundation, Rockefeller Foundation, Harvard University, the State Department, real estate agencies, and the like. The merger of agencies also brought to India and other Point four programs individuals from European programs, some excellent, some not so good, generally accustomed to more formal organizational procedures, some disgruntled because of a loss in pay and diplomatic passport incurred in the transfer, and some who looked upon TCA types as being soft-headed "do-gooders."

India

While India did not become involved in mutual security or defense support programs, recruitment and contracting for the delivery of American technical specialists suffered from the reorganization in Washington. An airgram Fritz had sent Washington on December 15, 1952 had led to the arrival in India the following summer of about 30 engineering professors from the universities of Illinois and Wisconsin. But after the reorganization Fritz found it very difficult to locate anyone in Washington who could provide a status report on the recruitment and contracting of over 100 technical specialists needed in India although they had been requested many months earlier on the special forms required.

Morale and study group

During the late 1950s under the International Cooperation Administration, a real effort was made to improve the morale of employees. Certain types of positions were expected to be in long-term demand, and officers in those categories were offered career opportunities. The President's Report on foreign aid of 1959 also set forth the proposition that technical assistance was a long-term program based on needs which would continue for the remainder of the century. The report called for a major study into the problems and processes of technical assistance which would enable the United States to improve its TA programs.

The author was assigned to the study group during 1960-61. The group carried out hundreds of interviews, reviewed hundreds of reports, and made a real effort to classify its findings in a meaningful way. The study, however, made no impact on the program. The prestigious social scientist planned to head the study was never hired. As the Eisenhower administration came to a close, it was perhaps too much to expect that a prestigious social scientist would risk his reputation on something which might be thrown out by the succeeding administration. After the election, the administration considered itself as being in a lame duck position, which it was, and stopped recruitment efforts. A later call on a high official of President Kennedy's administration elicited the response that the study indeed was important, but not of highest priority; therefore, recruitment of the social scientist would be put on the back burner. The inevitable result was that the study group withered away; its "bright young men" found other jobs.

President Kennedy's initial pronouncements and actions on foreign aid were generally greeted with favor by the insiders of the principal foreign economic aid organization of the time, the International Cooperation Administration, but he could have done nothing more harmful to employee morale than to announce publicly that he was seeking 50 executives from private business to head his overseas aid missions. It was true, of course, that duds could be found among ICA mission directors; there also were some very good ones, and the agency had plenty of good men and women waiting in the wings for positions of higher responsibility. Nevertheless, the administration went ahead with "Operation Tycoon." Some of the recruits were duds also, but thankfully most of them left within two or three years and presumably returned to more lucrative positions in private enterprise. One of the best stayed on and currently holds a top position in AID.

The administration also made it clear that it, too, desired a large reduction in force. President Kennedy's first administrator proved a bit lenient on this score and was relieved. The second administrator proved tougher. A great deal of uncertaintly ensued during a rather lengthy process. A number of responsible officers and their families were left stranded in overseas posts while their cases were reviewed in Washington; meanwhile their ability to work with the local government had been displaced by the mark of distrust demonstrated by the United States government. Their usefulness had been destroyed.

AID's creation

Meanwhile, several outside task forces had been recruited to do a quick job of examining the existing agency and programs and to devise new legislation and a new organization. Outsiders were brought in to head all the bureaus created in the new Agency for International Development (AID). The task forces made a point of avoiding discussion with senior executives of the old agency. No one looked at the findings of the Technical Assistance study group, and the meaning of technical assistance almost disappeared with invention of a new nomenclature, "development grants." Airgrams sent to all missions requested the submission of new programs based on the "turn-around" philosophy and pending legislation. While the "old hands" found it difficult to challenge the "transitional" programs which were submitted, judging that the missions still knew their countries better than they, some of the new hands were not timid about deleting whole pages of program presentations, sometimes without reading them.

Following these events was a long process of codifying policy and procedures for the new agency, AID. The author was heavily engaged in this process. The really powerful bureaus were the geographic bureaus which employed their own personnel and contracting staff as well as technical experts and generalists. But within broad limits, they were free to develop their own policies and procedures, and these became a hodgepodge after a few years. And while there was much lip service given to the delegation of responsibility to field missions, some bureaus were more intent on demanding reports for testimony to Congressman Passman than in delegating power and responsibility to mission directors on the scene. The one exception to the power position of the geographic bureaus was the strong position of the Office of Public Safety. While public safety and internal security programs reached their zenith of unpopularity in later years, few remembered that they were given their original impetus during the Kennedy administration.

After a settling down period, the agency performed reasonably well for a few years, perhaps a bit too bureaucratic, but nevertheless it functioned. It was responsible for a broad range of programs, both loans and grants for agriculture, health, education, private enterprise, public safety, food aid, disaster relief, and security supporting assistance.

Reorganization

Then in the late sixties several new events occurred. Two new reductions in force were conducted, one called BALPA, to designate the savings to occur in the United States balance of payments, and the other OPRED, or Operation Reduction. Both involved contractual as well as direct hire reductions, and they had to be accomplished by hasty reprogramming exercises, but a countering buildup of programs and personnel took place in Southeast Asia during the late sixties. Employees morally unwilling to go to Vietnam left the agency, and many new AID people in Vietnam turned out to be early military retirees.

A new reorganization also occurred during the late sixties when the agency decided to centralize some of its staff functions, including personnel and contracting staff, engineers, and auditors. The auditors were first removed from mission control and centralized in a Washington staff; later they were placed in regionally located offices of the AID auditor general. The personnel, contracting, and engineering staff were removed from the geographic bureaus and placed in a Bureau for Administration.

As years went on, initially mission loan officers were reassigned to Washington, then more and more technical and administrative people. Mission directors responded to Washington's requests to reduce staff more enthusiastically than anticipated. Many returnees to Washington filled unauthorized positions because the agency was not yet ready for another reduction in force, but then the ax fell. Thousands of personnel returned from Laos and Vietnam, and something had to be done. A mass reduction in force therefore took place in 1974-75. It included all public safety people and all personnel who were on limited appointment as well as others. Early retirements were actively encouraged. Following several years of attrition in AID staffing, the total effect was a decrease from 18,000 direct-hire employees in the late 1960s to 6,056 in 1976. (5)

Technical Assistance Bureau

Meanwhile, during the mid-1970s, an AID bureau in Washington called the Technical Assistance Bureau (TAB) began to grow. Its principal functions were to provide scientific leadership in each of the technical areas like agriculture, nutrition, education and health; to conduct an R and D program; and to support the geographic bureaus and overseas missions when special technical expertise was needed. The director of the Office of Agriculture reported after an overseas trip that the missions' agricultural staffs were so denuded that there were few people with whom he could communicate effectively. Other technical officers reported in a similar vein.

The AID organization of geographic bureaus was based on the sound premise that the USAID missions abroad were most qualified to assess the needs and capabilities of the countries in which they worked and that the corresponding country desk officers of AID in Washington were most qualified to communicate such assessments to policy makers. The weakening of USAIDs and the buildup of specialized Washington bureaus served to dilute this premise.

In TAB, for example, there were some people with little or no experience in overseas programs who were not convinced of the need to obtain USAID support or participation for research work in a specific country. There were other old overseas hands working in the bureau, who because of agency trends considered that initiation and control of programs from AID in Washington were the "wave of the future."

On the other hand, many AID recipient governments had established over the years, often with local USAID encouragement, central agencies responsible for coordinating matters of foreign aid. These were intended to assure that developmental priorities, local budget resources, and most suitable external aid resources were considered in accordance with rules that those governments deemed most appropriate. USAID officers knew and understood these rules; Washington-based officers did not. On occasion a TAB contractor selected a particular country in which to promote a research effort of international significance. Sometimes the particular country had not yet determined that it should play such a role. On some occasions contractors did not understand or follow the local rules or engage the local USAID adequately in going about their business. Under such conditions, if TAB at the last moment of decision making informed USAID of the country's selection and requested "country clearance," one should not be too surprised at a resultant flap.

Some AID officers have suggested that some of the problems which arose in this case study, particularly the jeep problem related in Cahpter 6, arose out of just such a flap. How could USAID do any better if HKI worked out the whole program with TAB, then at the last minute realized it had a problem and that only USAID/Jakarta could help? Understanding the prevalence of the syndrome and USAID's helpful attitudes, the author was willing to concede the point. Further examination of the record shows, however, that HKI's director of Blindness Prevention kept USAID officers fully informed of the project in its formative stages, as well as the need for jeeps; thus, USAID was preparing procurement documentation some months before the project got underway.

AID staffing.

Returning to agency trends and the denuding of USAID mission technical staff, even the agency's deputy administrator opined at a 1975 staff meeting that mission staff reductions had gone a bit too far; perhaps there should be some movement in the other direction. About six months later, he noted that despite his previous suggestion mission staff levels continued to decline. He was advised that his suggestion had never been conveyed to the mission directors who were continuing to follow old orders.

In the New York Times of February 26, 1978, the present administrator of AID, former Governor Gilligan of Ohio, is quoted as saying that the personnel of the agency is "overaged, overpaid and over here" and the Front Lines of January 5, 1978 reported that another agency RIF (reduction in force) "may become unavoidable."

It must be admitted that the agency had grown top heavy. Part of the problem was natural. If an agency expects to provide expert assistance around the world, it should have a cadre of experts who tend to be older and higher paid than average technicians. The other part of the problem, however, was a direct reflection of the events previously described. (6) Good young people were discouraged by the reorganizations, changing policies and procedures, reductions in force, the lack of opportunity for advancement in the face of continuing incursions by high ranking outsiders, and the general growing unpopularity of the organization. Despite attempts to encourage recruitment of young people through competition for internships, the author has seen graduates of such internships lose their jobs during the next reduction in force. And can anyone blame the older people who are hanging on long enough to earn their retirement credentials?

Congressional input

The Congress has not been derelict in its attention to the agency. Its committees have held lengthy hearings and demanded volumes of information. Congress has amended and reamended the basic legislation. It has imposed increasing restrictions upon the agency's operations. Some Congressmen like security supporting assistance and despise economic aid; others prefer options that are vice versa. Many have their own favorite countries. Some want the agency to support human rights and others to support United States military allies. Some favor health, and others favor education. It is difficult to run an agency with broad international responsibilities in a manner which will satisfy all Congressmen. If AID is a monster, it is a monster that has been created and evolved by succeeding Congresses and administrations; it is a monster they deserve.

FUTURE AGENDA

Perhaps it is too late. Perhaps there is no cure. Perhaps we should dump the whole mess. Perhaps it isn't worth the bother.

The author's view is that failure to cooperate decently with other democratic countries in helping the poorer countries is a failure the American government and people must not accept. It is not the function of this case study to prove that provision of such help is in America's interest; that function is being performed very well by publications of the Overseas Development Council, the World Watch Institute, and others. But the author is convinced that the United States must continue its foreign aid and that it must do a better job.

As this final chapter is being written, the United States Congress is considering a bill which proposes another "sweeping reorganization in the administration of foreign aid." (7) The author recognizes the responsibility of any foreign aid agency to the president and to the Congress and that organization of the agency must reflect that responsibility. At the same time, the author is hopeful that such an organization will also recognize the realities of the technical assistance process. The overriding concern of the agency in the past has been its survival in the face of congressional onslaughts, but too much concern with survival is likely to damage an organization's ability to act. (8)

AID is an extremely complex organization with multifaceted functions relating to a multitude of programs scattered around many countries in every continent except Australia and Antarctica. The agency called for in the bill currently under consideration will be even more complex. The common bond throughout the AID organization and its programs is a high degree of uncertainty. The new organization will not change in this respect. It might be well to examine what current social science literature has to say about the subject. A massive review of the literature sets forth the following relevant contention:

> Organizations that operate under conditions of high degree of certainty (internally or externally) tend to be characterized by centralization in decision making. Further, this relationship is associated with efficiency of operation. Conversely, where there are relatively high degrees of uncertainty, modes of operation and effectiveness are associated with decentralization in decision making. (9)

The study finds strong support in the literature for this contention and no studies in opposition. (10) It also states that a well-established base of theory lends credence to the generalization. It concludes that "practitioners in organizations functioning under relatively high degrees of uncertainty should consider decentralized structural arrangements in order to increase effectiveness."

The author has hinted strongly during this case study that responsibility and decision making should be located as closely as possible to the scene of action, where the changes take place, where the people involved feel most concerned, and where it is more likely that solutions can be undertaken rapidly and effectively. He is gratified to find the following quotation to support this thesis:

> Research findings also suggest that where there is a high degree of uncertainty, decision-making that is decentralized or shared among different levels in the organization is conducive to effectiveness. In this situation, knowledge is not easily concentrated at higher levels of the organization, since environmental factors are in flux. Thus, units of the organization directly in touch and dealing with the changing conditions are best equipped to react quickly and make, or share in the making of, decisions. (11)

If one were to follow this logically, he would have assigned all commodity procurement responsibility in the Vitamin A Blindness Research Project to HKI, and the slit lamp, cameras, typewriters,

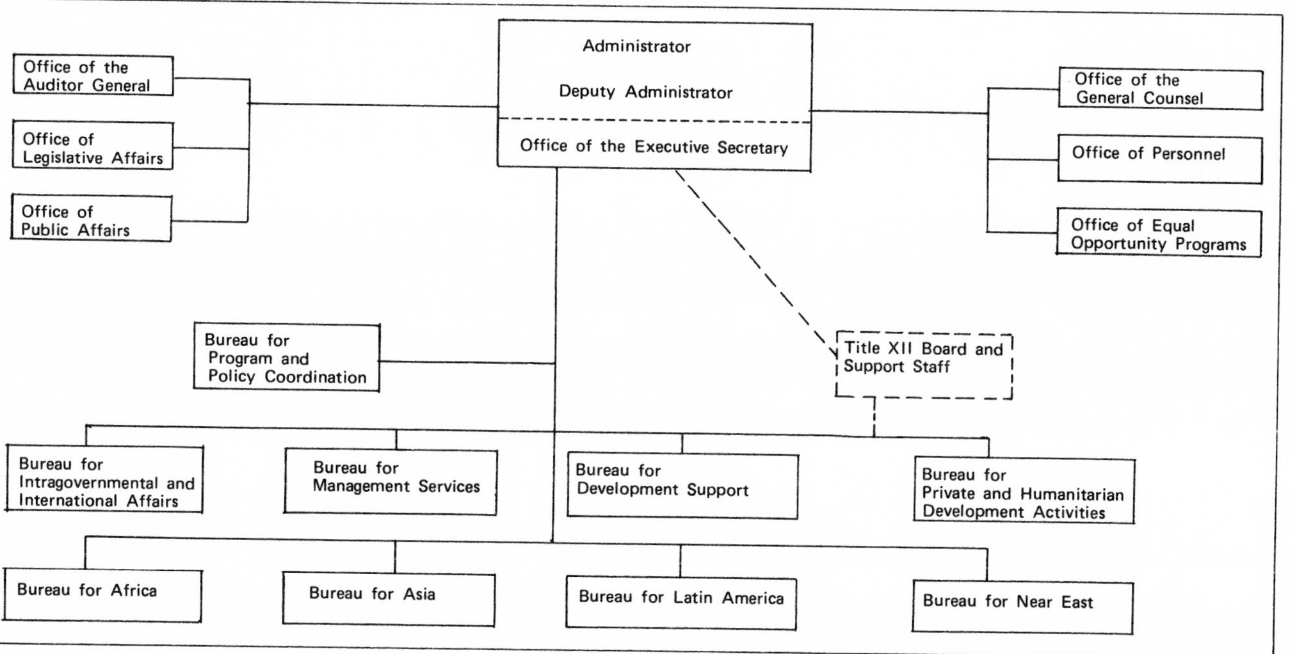

Fig. 11.1. AID reorganization proposed by its organization task force.

Source: Front Lines, November 17, 1978.

and jeeps would have arrived on time, or headquarters would have heard directly from its employees on the job.

But this is a bit naive. United States government procurement procedures are rather complicated, and HKI is not a procurement agency. It might have violated AID and federal procurement regulations trying to be one. While procurement regulations are quite complex, they contain no high degree of uncertainty. Procedures must be followed meticulously and expertly. If the responsible officer is far from the scene of action and if he has a sizeable workload, he will perform the job in the routine which suits him and his immediate superiors best. And this kind of organizational pattern is most congenial to officers in such positions. Thus, a procurement order for jeeps issued by USAID in Jakarta in October 1976 was reissued by AID in Washington in March 1977. The principal change was the notation that "This authorization has been reviewed and approved in accordance with the President's Memorandum of September 16, 1966, concerning economy in procurement." If the officer responsible had been located in USAID in Jakarta, he would have received pressure from project officers in Bandung. If he had been located in the same office or bureau with the AID in Washington desk officer for Indonesia, he might have received some pressure to move the document, but in this case he was far removed organizationally from the scene of action, the area of environmental change, the source of pressure, and he felt no need to deviate from his routine.

The same principle applies to personnel officers, contract officers, loan officers, engineers, and technical specialists. When they are located in the AID field mission or Washington's geographical bureau, they have a more direct interest in the problem under discussion, feel greater responsibility toward the mission, and find greater pressure exerted upon them for action. But, someone will ask: who will integrate these functions when the experts are scattered around the geographical bureaus and overseas missions, who assures agency-wide agriculture policy, who assures that procurement and contract regulations and procedures are followed and modified as the basic legislation is changed; and who puts the whole picture together for outside audiences like the Congress?

In an agency as large as AID, there is always room for a special office or offices dealing with policy and management procedures. And in such a special office, why should the agency not locate some of its best brains to perform these functions? They can receive periodic reports from their counterparts in the geographic bureaus who are closer to the changing circumstances. They can meet regularly to work out improved policies and procedures which are realistic in terms of the uncertain conditions which exist. If visitors cannot find the person responsible for a particular function, these specialists can steer them in the right direction.

One of the problems with past reorganizations has been their episodic and violent nature. Such efforts inevitably array the advocates of reorganization (generally outsiders) against the inside defenders of the status quo. They have a traumatic effort on the agency's employees. But in the view of a distinguished public administrator, the more significant reorganizations come from incremental changes brought about by continuous internal pressure. (12) It was gratifying to note in the Front Lines of November 17, 1977 that the latest AID organization task force recommended an "evolutionary rather than revolutionary decentralization to avoid undue disruption and damage to morale and to preserve and enhance program effectiveness." The report also noted the shortages of personnel in the technical development disciplines. It also suggested that AID be divorced from security supporting assistance. All of these recommendations tend to coincide with the author's views. However, it takes more than reorganization to change an agency like AID. It requires clearly stated, defensible goals; a basic change in attitude; a conversion of prevalent cynicism; and a rededication to the ideals for which the agency stands. All of these require leadership which possesses the confidence of the president and the Congress and an ability to instill the desired changes of attitude in the agency's employees; a certain security of tenure; and reassurance by the Congress that foreign aid and technical assistance are continuing instruments of long-term foreign policy and are not to be diverted to short-term political ends.

Perhaps all of these requirements are too much to ask, but if the United States wants to regain in the eyes of the world its lost promise of leadership in those international affairs which mean so much for the future of the world we live in, its deeds will speak louder than words.

The late, indomitable Senator Humphrey really said it all in his introduction to the International Development Cooperation Act of 1978, which he said was designed to address three fundamental issues:

> First,...we are out to assist the poorest people to overcome the worst aspects of absolute poverty.
>
> Second,...we want to remove all legislative and administrative restrictions that do not advance this goal.
>
> Third,...we need to organize ourselves administratively to accomplish this goal. (13)

Appendix 1

Agreement between the Government of Indonesia
and
the American Foundation for Overseas Blind

Concerning the Characterization of Vitamin A Deficiency and Xerophthalmia in Indonesia and the Design of Effective Intervention Programs.

Introduction

Recognizing that the lack of vitamin A nutrient in the diet is a threat of blindness and ill health to a significant number of preschool children, the Government of the Republic of Indonesia (hereinafter to be referred to as the Government) initiated a two year pilot project of distribution of massive dose vitamin A capsules in 20 subdistricts in Java. The American Foundation for Overseas Blind (AFOB) entered into an agreement with the Government in March 1973 to provide technical assistance and funds for indigenous personnel required for the evaluation of the effectiveness of delivery system.

Based on this experience and the evaluation finding the development of alternate interventions for prevention and control of vitamin A deficiency caused blindness are indicated. AFOB made available an expert in the field of epidemiology and of ophthalmology, Dr. Alfred Sommer of Johns Hopkins University, for two months in 1975 to serve as a Consultant to the Ministry of Health in developing a plan to obtain facts as to magnitude and geographical distribution of the prevalence of vitamin A deficiency and to identify the causative factors and characteristics of the population at highest risk of blindness from the vitamin deficiency.

Based on the above mentioned evaluation finds the Ministry of Health proposed to make adjustments in the vitamin A intervention program to be carried out during PELITA II so that there will be a better appreciation of all the factors necessary for implementing an effective and efficient program during PELITA III. This project, commencing in August 1976 and concluding by July 1979, will be carried out in cooperation with the Directorate General of Community Health and the National Institute of Health Research and Development. AFOB is prepared to provide an expert scientist, Dr. Sommer, to give technical guidance and participate with the Indonesian staff in the project's implementation. He is available for residence in Indonesia for the duration of the project. The administration, management, and research activities will be the responsibility of the concerned Indonesian Authorities although a substantial proportion of the costs will be covered by the AFOB.

Now, therefore the Government and AFOB have entered into the following agreement for the implementation of the proposed project which is designed to make a major contribution to the prevention of blindness in Indonesian children.

Article I

The basic objectives of the project are (a) to establish the magnitude and geographic distribution of vitamin A related blindness in children in Indonesia; (b) define epidemiologically (mild) xerophthalmia and (severe) keratomalacia in order to identify those factors responsible for their occurrence and amenable to effective intervention; (c) utilize these findings in the design of national intervention programs for prevention and control of blinding disease in children in particular and other related disease in children caused by vitamin A deficiency.

The project is devided into four integrated studies, managed and coordinated by a central, supporting unit. West Java has been selected for the location, with operations centered in Bandung.

Article II

Responsibilities of AFOB

AFOB will assist the Government in the development of the design for the studies and in their implementation and planning for action oriented solution to the problem of vitamin A deficiency based on the study findings. Specifically, AFOB will:

1. Provide the services of a qualified expert in epidemiology and ophthalmology, Dr. Alfred Sommer, for the duration of the project.

2. Provide funds to supplement salaries of Indonesian staff to compensate for heavy responsibility and intensive work effort during the project.

3. Provide or be instrumental in the provision of agreed upon equipment and transport needed to effectively carry out the operation.

4. Underwrite necessary computer costs for data analysis if facilities are not available within the Government.

5. Make available the service of an AFOB project liaison officer to carry out liaison functions between AFOB in New York and the responsible project officials and the Government.

Article III

Responsibilities of the Government

The head of the National Institute of Health Research and Development will serve as the project director and in conjunction with the director general of Community Health, will appoint a steering committee to serve in advisory capacity to the project staff and scientist. Specifically, the Government will:

1. Provide without charge suitable space and office furniture needed for effective operation in the Bandung area, and communication services including telephone, postage, and cable.

2. For data gathering and analysis, provision will be made for printed questionnaire forms, card punching, and if available from the facilities of the Ministry of Health, the computerized programs.

3. Select and made available to work on the project for the duration of their assignment the supporting staff and the research

team personnel including the ophthalmologists, pediatricians, nutritionists, and nurses required with supplementary per diem and transport costs.

Article IV

General Provisions

In accordance with the law and regulations enforced in Indonesia:

1. The Government will provide certificates of residence and work permits for the AFOB scientist and project liaison officer and their respective families.

2. All payment to the AFOB scientist and liaison officer shall be exempted to the extent permitted by laws from any taxation which may now or hereinafter be imposed thereon by laws of the Government.

3. The Government shall accord exemption from custom duty and from other fees and charges, if any, relating to all equipment, materials, and supplies imported into Indonesia for the purpose of performing services under this agreement.

4. No custom duties shall be imposed by the Government with respect to any equipment, materials, or supplies imported into Indonesia as food or personal belongings of AFOB personnel, for the use of that personnel, either at the approximate time of the personnel's arrival, or at a later date during the personnel's period of residence within Indonesia.

5. The Government will allow AFOB to purchase some vehicles needed for the project from local assembly plants.

6. AFOB scientist and liaison officer and their dependents will be granted "Bebas Bea" visas and permission to leave and reenter the country.

7. After consultation with the head of the National Institute of Health Research and Development, AFOB may send their officers and executives to Indonesia as may be required to view the progress of the work; traveling costs and allowances will be borne by AFOB.

Article V

Final Provisions

1. The detailed plan of operation of the proposed project is attached, and any alterations or amendments shall be determined by the Government and AFOB by mutual consent.

2. This agreement shall enter into force commencing 1976 and shall remain in effect during the period of three years, concluding June 1979.

3. This agreement will be effective as of 1976 and shall bind each party hereto and shall continue to be in force until June 30, 1979, provided, however, that this agreement may be terminated at any time by either party upon transmission to and receipt by the other party of 90 days written notice.

4. This agreement is done in English in four originals, this 30th day of August 1976.

In witness whereof, the undersigned, being duly authorized have signed this agreement.

For the Government of the Republic of Indonesia

Djaka Sutadiwiria
Secretary General
Ministry of Health

For the American Foundation for Overseas Blind

Alfred Sommer M. D.
Project Scientist

Appendix 2

Proyex Penanggulangan Kebutaan
Jl. Cicendo No. 4
Bandung

Manual for Completion Form 103
Form 103A
Family
Baseline Census - Survey

Definitions and Instructions

A single form 103A should be completed on each family. The enumerator should interview the most knowledgeable member of the family. All notations should be "right justified." A family is defined as all individuals who live under the same roof and eat out of the same cooking pot.

I. Family Identification

1. Form number: this form is already precoded: 1   1

2. Study number: this form is already precoded: number: 100   2, 3, 4

3. Village code number: 01 = Citalang   5, 6
   02 = Karoya
   03 = Cikao Bandung

04 = Cilegong
05 = Kembangkuning
06 = Cisarua
07 =
08 =
09 =
10 =

4. R. K. Code number: 7, 8

5. R. T. Code number: 9, 10

6. House number: this will be assigned sequentially; the first house in each R. T. getting the number 1 11, 12

7. Family number: there may be more than one family (defined as all individuals eating out of the same cooking pot whether or not they are blood relatives). This includes the nuclear family, other relatives, servants who live with the family, long-term visitors, and anyone else who is spending at least two months more as a part of the family. The first family in that house will be numbered 1, the second family number 2, etc. 13

8. Team number: this is the code number assigned to each enumerator. See separate list. 14, 15

9. Name of the head of household: this should be written into the appropriate space. There is no column assigned to this. The head of the family is that individual who is responsible for managing the family's budget. If the husband is available, he should be the head of the family. If it is a wife who is separated or widowed, she is then the head of the family.

10. Date of the interview.
    - Day. 16, 17
    - Month. 18, 19
    - Year. 20, 21

11. Was the family interviewed? 22
    1 = yes
    2 = no, because they were not at home.
    3 = no, because they were not cooperative.
    4 = no, for other reasons.

12. List the number of individuals residing in this family. 23, 24

13. Number of children under six years of age residing in that family. This includes all children whether or not they are blood relatives of the family (infants, orphans, step-children, long-term guests, servant's children, etc). 25

II. Economic and Social Information of the Family

1. What is the major source of income (in money or kind) for this family? 26
    1 = entirely agricultural
    2 = entirely non agricultural
    3 = mixture of agricultural and non agricultural, but agricultural being the most inportant
    4 = mixture of agricultural and non agricultural, but non agricultural being the most important

2. Number of adult livestock owned by the family:
    chicken and ducks 27, 28, 29
    sheeps and goats 30, 31
    cows and buffalos 32, 33
    horses 34
    pigs 35, 36

3. Does the family own one or more fish ponds: A fish pond is defined as a pool of water at least 5 x 5 m, in which fish are grown: 37
    1 = yes
    2 = no

4. The most expensive material used in the construction of the walls of the house: 38
    1 = brick

2 = wood
3 = bamboo
4 = other

5. The most expensive material used in the construction of the floor of the house: 39
   1 = tile
   2 = cement
   3 = wood
   4 = bamboo
   5 - dirt
   6 = other

6. Source of lighting house at night: 40
   1 = electricity
   2 = gas lantern
   3 = oil lamp
   4 = other
   5 = none
   6 = do not know

7. Source of drinking water: 41
   1 = pipe water supply into the house
   2 = hand or electric pump (closed well)
   3 = private open well
   4 = general open well
   5 = surface water
   6 = river water
   7 = rain water
   8 = other

8. Bathing place regardless of source of water 42
   1 = bathroom within the house
   2 = bathroom shared with the general public not within the house
   3 = other

III. <u>Items eaten by the family</u>

1. The major staple food eaten during the past harvest season: 43
   1 = rice
   2 = cassava

3 = corn
4 = sweet potato
5 = other

2. Main staple food consumed by family during the period preceding the past harvest season: 44
   1 = rice
   2 = cassava
   3 = corn
   4 = sweet potato
   5 = other

3. Which of the following did the family harvest for their own consumption during the six months preceding the past harvest season? 1 = yes 2 = no
   Rice 45
   Cassava 46
   Corn 47
   Sweet potato 48
   Vegetable 49
   Fruit 50

Appendix 3

Form 103B: Individual
Base Line Census Survey

Definition and Instructions	Column
A single form 103B should be filled out on every member of the family (people living under the same roof and eating out of the same cooking pot whether or not they are blood relatives). Certain questions pertain to only certain members of the family. These are noted on the form. The questions should be asked of the most knowledgeable members of the family.	
I. Identification numbers	
1. Form number: this is already self-coded as: 2	1
2. Study number: this is already self-coded as: 100	2, 3, 4
3. Village number: these are the same as for form 103A	5, 6
4. RK code number: these are the same as on form 103A	7, 8
5. RT code number: these are the same as on form 103A	9, 10

6. House code number: same as form 103A 11, 12

7. Family number: same as form 103A 13

8. Individual identification number: each individual should have a separate form 103B, and be assigned their own sequential identification number. The first individual (number 01) should be the head of the household. This is the individual responsible for arranging all financial matters in that family. The remaining individuals should be listed in the following order: spouse, children, including stepchildren (eldest first), other relatives, nonrelatives. 14, 15

9. Name of the individual: simply write in the person's name. This is not coded for IBM punching.

10. Age of the individual:

    a. All children under the age of 6 should have their exact date of birth recorded in either the Islamic or International calendar. Write in the month and the year of birth. Use the conversion chart to fill in the exact age in months completed. If the date of birth is not known by either calendar method, enter digits 99. 16, 17

    b. The age in years completed. This should be completed on all members of the family whether or not they are under the age of 6. 18, 19

11. Sex: 1 = male 2 = female 20

12. Does the individual have difficulty getting about the village during the daylight hours because of poor vision? This is defined as requiring some aid, either another individual, a dog or a stick. 21
    1 = yes 2 = no 3 = do not know

II. Educational Studies

1. The highest certificate obtained (school completed). 22
   1 = did not attend school or did not finish primary school
   2 = Primary school
   3 = Junior high school
   4 = Senior high school
   5 = Academy
   6 = University
   9 = do not know

2. Total number of years of schooling (highest class attended): 23, 24
   If the answer is unknown enter the digits 99.

III. The following information is gathered only on females 12 years or older.

1. Number of children under the age of 6 residing in that family that they have given birth to. If they have given birth to no children put number 0. 25

IV. The following information is inquired only of those women who have children residing in the family under the age of six to whom they have given birth.

1. Marital status. 26
   1 = not yet married. 2 = the first wife of the first marriage and still married to that original husband. 3 = the first wife of an additional marriage (second, third, etc.) and still living with the husband of the last marriage. 4 = first wife of the last marriage (may be first, second, third, etc. marriage), but widowed, separated, or divorced from the last husband. 5 = second wife (or third or fourth wife) and still married to her first husband. 6 = a second wife (or lower) who has remarried and is living with the last husband. 7 = a second wife as above, but either separated, divorced, or widowed. 9 = do not know.

2. Age of the woman at the time of her first marriage. 27
1 = Less than 16 years of age. 2 = 16–19 years.
3 = 20–24 years. 4 = 25–29 years. 5 = 30–34 years.
6 = 35–39 years. 7 = older than age 39.

3. Number of live births to this woman. This is defined as any child who showed any sign of life at the time of birth, regardless of whether or not he subsequently died. 28, 29

4. Number of children who are still alive at the present time and were born to this woman. 30, 31

5. Number of children born to this woman who subsequently died. This is the difference between numbers 4 and 5 above. 32

V. The following information pertains only to <u>children under the age of 6</u>.

1. Enter the code number of the individual who actually feeds the child and takes care of him. 33, 34

2. Relationship of this individual to the child. 35
1 = mother. 2 = grandmother. 3 = sister.
4 = brother. 5 = aunt. 6 = close relative.
7 = other. 9 = do not know.

3. 3. Which parents of this child live in the house as part of the family? 1 = original father. 36
2 = original mother. 3 = father and mother.
4 = neither.

4. What other relatives are members of the family? 1 = grandmother or grandfather. 37
2 = other adult close relatives. 3 = both.
4 = neither.

VI. The following questions pertain only to those individuals over the age of 12.

1. What is the major source of income in money or kind? 1 = all agricultural. 2 = all nonagricultural. 3 = mixed, but mostly agricultural. 4 = mixed but mostly nonagricultural. 38

2. What is the main source of income from agricultural work? 1 = farm owner. 2 = share cropper. 3 = owner and share cropper. 4 = rent land. 5 = laborer. 6 = perennial crops. 39

3. What is the main source of income from nonagricultural work? 1 = government official. 2 = itinerant salesman. 3 = factory or shop owner. 4 = crafts. 5 = professional. 6 = laborer. 7 = servant. 8 = other. 40

NUTRITIONAL BLINDNESS
PREVENTION PROJECT

PROYEK PENANGGULANGAN KEBUTAAN

JL. CICENDO 4--BANDUNG

Form 104
Family Registration Card
Kartu Registrasi Keluarga

IDENTITY

1. Village name	No.
2. RK#	
3. RT#	
4. House number	
5. Family number	
6. Head of family	
7. Name of supervisor	

Group: CHILDREN UNDER 6 YEARS OLD																			
				Number and date of exam															
No.	Child's Name	Age	Sex	1	2	3	4	5	6	7	8	9	10	11	12	13	14	15	16
SUPERVISOR'S SIGNATURE																			

APPENDIX 4

Form 106
Census Book

Village________________ No. R.K._____ No. R.T._____ No. House_____ No. Family_____

					Number and date of examination																
No.	Family members	Age	Sex	Person caring for child	1	2	3	4	5	6	7	8	9	10	11	12	13	14	15	16	Remarks
1.																					
2.																					
3.																					
4.																					
5.																					
6.																					
7.																					
8.																					
9.																					
10.																					
11.																					
12.																					
13.																					
14.																					

APPENDIX 5

Notes

PREFACE

1. Robert Morris, "Community Planning for Health: The Social Welfare Experience," in Public Health Concepts in Social Work Education, Council on Social Work Education, 1962, pp. 168-9.

CHAPTER 1

1. Dr. Marcus Ingle agrees that changes in plans will become necessary as the project proceeds and states "that this agrees with everything I found in the literature" (personal communication, 1978).

2. J. G. Bauernfeind, "Vitamin A Technology and Xerophthalmia" (Report to Office of Nutrition, Agency for International Development: Washington, D. C., 1973), p. 1.

3. For the material in this section the author has drawn heavily on a 1977 publication of Helen Keller International, "The Right to See." This publication is furnished free of charge by Helen Keller International Inc., 22 West 17th Street, New York, N. Y. 10011, U. S. A.

4. Nick Cole, Gemini News Service, "World Moves to Give Sight to Millions," Times of Indonesia, July 25, 1978.

5. Ibid.

6. Assistance for Blind Children, Bulletin One (Dacca, Bangladesh, August 31, 1978).

7. "Xerophthalmia Group" (Report of the First Assembly-International Agency for the Prevention of Blindness, Oxford, July 5-9, 1978).

8. Andre G. Van Veen and Marjorie Scott Van Veen, "Vitamin A Problems with Special Reference to Less Developed Countries" (Report to Office of Nutrition, Agency for International Development, Washington, D. C., 1973).

9. Solon, Fernandez, and Popkin, "Research to Determine the Cost and Effectiveness of Alternate Means of Controlling Vitamin A Deficiency, and an Evaluation of Three Alternate Strategies to Prevent Xerophthalmia in the Philippines" (Cornell University, 1977), p. 30 of appendix. The authors cite Jogjakarta, Indonesia where a Dutch physician, Professor Oomen, collected 11,000 xerophthalmia case histories from free clinics, but not one while scanning thousands of records of paying patients.

10. International Vitamin A Consultative Group, Guidelines for the Eradication of Vitamin A Deficiency and Xerophthalmia (New York: Nutrition Foundation, 1976), p. III-1.

11. Van Veen and Van Veen, "Vitamin A Problems," p. 21.

12. AID project paper of 1975.

13. Helen Keller, 1952, quoted in "HKI Report, January 1-June 30, 1976."

CHAPTER 2

1. Jack Rothman, Planning and Organizing for Social Change (New York: Columbia University Press, 1974), p. 30.

2. American Foundation for the Overseas Blind, "Evaluation of the Vitamin A Deficiency Prevention Pilot Project in Indonesia," (New York, 1975).

3. "Vitamin A Deficiency and Xerophthalmia," WHO Technical Report Series, No. 590 (Report of a Joint WHO/USAID Meeting, Geneva, 1976).

4. "A Proposal for the Characterization of Vitamin A Deficiency and Xerophthalmia in Indonesia, A Basis for the Design of Effective Intervention Programs" (Report prepared for the Ministry of Health, Government of Indonesia, and the American Foundation for the Overseas Blind, New York, revised April 1976).

5. Memorandum from Chief, Scientific Programs Branch, United States National Eye Institute, National Institutes of Health, Washington, D. C., February 12, 1976.

CHAPTER 3

1. B. R. Burkhalter, "A Critical Review of Nutritional Planning Models and Experience," Community Systems Foundation, for Office of Nutrition, AID, 1974, p. 36.

2. Dennis A. Rodinelli, "Implementing Development Projects: The Problem of Management," Focus: Technical Cooperation (Washington, D. C.: Society for International Development, 1978/1), p. 9.

3. Manoff International Inc., "Using Modern Marketing Techniques for Nutrition Education" (Report to AID on an experimental demonstration project in Ecuador, Washington, D. C., 1975), p. 15.

CHAPTER 4

1. Van Veen and Van Veen, "Vitamin A Problems," p. 47.

2. Manoff International Inc., "Using Modern Marketing Techniques for Nutrition Education" (Washington, D. C.: AID, 1975), p. 17.

3. On-site Review Team, Review of Government of Indonesia and American Foundation for Overseas Blind Project, "Characterization of Vitamin A Deficiency and Xerophthalmia in Indonesia - A

Basis for the Design of Effective Intervention Programs" (Washington, D. C.: AID, January 1977).

4. Burkhalter, "A Critical Review of Nutrition Planning Models," p. 92.

5. Meyer N. Zaid, Organizing for Community Welfare (Chicago: Quadrangle Books, 1967), p. 52, quoted in J. Rothman, Planning and Organizing for Social Change (New York: Columbia University Press, 1974), p. 63.

6. Rothman, Planning and Organizing for Social Change, p. 82.

CHAPTER 5

1. J. E. Austin, Global Malnutrition and Cereal Fortification (Report submitted by Harvard University to the United States Agency for International Development, 1977), p. 11.

CHAPTER 6

1. Burkhalter, "A Critical Review of Nutrition Planning Models," p. 62. This refers to a systems approach to nutrition planning in Tamil Nadu, India.

2. "Vitamin A Deficiency and Xerophthalmia," Technical Report Series, no. 590 (Report of a Joint WHO/USAID Meeting, World Health Organization, Geneva, 1976).

3. J. G. Sommer, Beyond Charity: U. S. Voluntary Aid for a Changing Third World (Washington, D. C.: Overseas Development Council, 1977), p. 102.

4. On-site Review Team, Review of Government of Indonesia and American Foundation for Overseas Blind Project, "Characterization of Vitamin A Deficiency and Xerophthalmia in Indonesia -- A Basis for the Design of Effective Intervention Programs" (Washington, D. C.: AID, January, 1977).

5. Burkhalter, "A Critical Review of Nutrition Planning Models," p. 53, citing conclusions from Alan Berg and Robert Muscat, The Nutritional Factor: Its Role in National Development (Washington, D. C., Brookings Institution).

6. Marcus Ingle, Program Implementation in Developing Countries (Report to AID Office of Development Administration, March 1978), p. 26.

CHAPTER 7

1. Jack Rothman, Planning and Organizing for Social Change, p. 125.

2. Sommer, Beyond Charity, p. 92.

3. Letter from Dr. Alfred Sommer to Dr. Susan T. Pettiss, October 11, 1976.

4. Letter from Dr. Susan T. Pettiss to Dr. Alfred Sommer, October 12, 1976.

CHAPTER 8

1. Van Veen and Van Veen, Vitamin A Problems, p. 32.

2. Indonesian Times, Jakarta, February 13, 1978.

CHAPTER 9

1. Francis C. Byrnes, "Role Shock: An Occupational Hazard of American Technical Assistants Abroad," The Annals of the American Academy of Political and Social Science, vol. 368, November 1966.

2. A foreign expert's comment cited in David Smith and Mabel Jessee, "Barriers between Expert and Counterpart," International Development Review, vol. 12, no. 1, 1970.

3. Jack Rothman, Planning and Organizing for Social Change, p. 40.

4. Kenneth Gerden and Mary Gerden, "What Other Nations Hear When the Eagle Screams." Psychology Today, June 1974, p. 54, quoted in John G. Sommer, Beyond Charity, p. 28.

5. Michael Roysten and Victor Jordan, "Self-Reliance and Environmental Management Education," Focus: Technical Cooperation, 1978/1, Society for International Development, Washington, D.C., p. 25.

6. A host country counterpart quoted in Smith and Jessee, "Barriers between Expert and Counterpart."

CHAPTER 10

1. F.J. Levinson and David L. Call, "Nutrition Intervention in Low Income Countries: A Planning Model and Case Study," Cornell International Agricultural Development, Mimeograph 34, 1970, p. 7; also J.C. Bauernfeind, "Vitamin A Technology," AID Office of Nutrition, 1973, pp. 74-75.

2. Latham, Solon, Fernandez, and Popkin, "Research to Determine the Cost and Effectiveness of Controlling Vitamin A Deficiency" and "Evaluation of Three Alternative Strategies to Prevent Xerophthalmia in the Philippines," Report to AID, 1977), p. 6.

3. Institute of Nutrition for Central America and Panama (INCAP), Fortification of Sugar with Vitamin A in Central America and Panama (Guatemala: INCAP, 1974), p. 4.

4. Nutritional Program Development in Indonesia, MIT International Nutrition Planning Program, Technical Report Series, no. 2, 1975.

5. Ibid., p. 23.

6. INCAP, Fortification of Sugar (AID financed the translation of this publication into English).

7. Albert Hirschman, Development Projects Observed (Washington, D.C.: The Brookings Institute, 1967), p. 11.

CHAPTER 11

1. N. Pattabhi Raman, "Project Implementation in the Context of a Plan: The Missing Links," Focus: Technical Cooperation, Washington, D.C.: Society for International Development, 1978/1, p. 4.

2. John D. Montgomery, The Politics of Foreign Aid, published for the Council on Foreign Relations (New York: Praeger, 1962), p. 151.

3. For example, see John D. Montgomery, The Politics of Foreign Aid; also see David A. Baldwin, Foreign AID and American Foreign Policy (New York: Praeger), 1966.

4. Ibid, p. 136.

5. "15 Years Later: A Quick Look Back," Front Lines (AID) 15, no. 1 (November 4, 1976): 6.

6. Thomas C. Niblock, "What to do about AID?" AID Forum, July 1978.

7. Ann Crittenden, "The Realpolitik of Foreign Aid," The New York Times, February 27, 1978.

8. Rothman, Planning and Organizing for Social Change, p. 140. This study was supported by a grant from the National Institute of Mental Health.

9. Ibid., pp. 29-30.

10. Rothman, ibid. The book cites the following research studies as being compatible with the proposition:

    M. Aiken and J. Hage, "Routine Technology, Social Structure and Organizational Goals," Administrative Science Quarterly 14, no. 3 (1969): 366-75.

R. Bar-Yosef and O. S. Schild. "Pressures and Defenses in Bureaucratic Rules," *American Journal of Sociology* 71, no. 6 (1966): 665-73.

S. R. Klatzky, "Organizational Size, Complexity and Coordination: Alternative Hypotheses" (Paper presented at American Sociological Association Meeting, San Francisco, 1969).

P. Lawrence and J. W. Lorsch, "Differentiation and Integration Coupled Organizations," *Administrative Science Quarterly* 12, no. 1 (1967), 1-47.

R. L. Simpson and W. H. Gullay, "Goals, Environmental Pressures and Organizational Characteristics," *American Sociological Review* 27, no. 3 (1962): 344-51.

H. Kauffman, *The Forest Ranger* (Baltimore: Johns Hopkins Press), 1960.

S. N. Eisenstadt and L. Katy, "Some Sociological Observations in the Response of Israeli Organizations to New Immigrants," *Administrative Science Quarterly* 5, no. 1 (1960): 113-33.

11. J. Rothman, *Planning and Organizing for Social Change*, p. 119.

12. Paul H. Appleby, "The Significance of the Hoover Commission Report," *Yale Review* 39, no. 1 (September 1949): 1-22.

13. As quoted in AID's *Front Lines* of February 16, 1978.

Glossary

AFOB	American Foundation for Overseas Blind, now known as Helen Keller International (HKI). Headquarters in New York City.
AID	Agency for International Development, the principal United States government foreign aid agency established in 1962. It inherited the role of several predecessor agencies by act of Congress. Its overseas missions are referred to as USAIDs.
BAPPENAS	The principal Indonesian government planning agency.
CP	Central examination points used by clinical and survey teams in this case study.
GSA	General Services Administration, a United States government agency which handles centralized procurement of commodities and purchase as well as lease and maintenance of government buildings.
HKI	Helen Keller International, formerly AFOB.
ICA	International Cooperation Administration, which administered United States foreign aid in the late 1950s up to 1961.
ITB	Institute of Technology, Bandung.

IU — International units.

IVACG — International Vitamin A Consultative Group. See Chapter 10.

MIT — Massachusetts Institute of Technology.

MSA — Mutual Security Agency established by legislation in 1951 as the successor to the Economic Cooperative Administration which administered Marshall Plan aid, mainly to Europe.

MSG — Monosodiumglutimate.

NEI — National Eye Institute, part of the United States National Institutes of Health, Bethesda, Maryland.

PIO/C — A Procurement Implementation Order/Commodities, an AID commodity procurement document.

PPUD — An Indonesian document needed for clearing official goods through Customs.

RBP — Retinal binding protein.

REPELITA — Indonesian initials for the five year plan.

SEKKAB — Secretary to the Government of Indonesia Cabinet.

TA — Technical assistance.

TCA — Technical Cooperation Administration, which administered point four assistance to developing countries in the early 1950s.

UNICEF — United Nations Children's Fund, New York City.

USAID — The overseas mission of AID, the Agency for International Development.

WHO — World Health Organization, a specialized agency of the United Nations, headquartered in Geneva, Switzerland.

Bibliography

Abelson, Philip H., ed. Food: Politics, Economics, Nutrition, and Research, American Association for the Advancement of Science. Washington, D. C.: 1975, p. 202.

AID. The AID Nutrition Program Strategy. Washington, D. C.: AID, 1973, p. 54.

AID. Front Lines, a biweekly internal news organ.

AID Evaluation Report. Review of Government of Indonesia and American Foundation for Overseas Blind Project, "Characterization of Vitamin A Deficiency and Xerophthalmia in Indonesia - A Basis for the Design of Effective Intervention Programs." Washington, D. C.: AID, January 1977.

AID. The Vitamin A Project in Indonesia. Washington, D. C.: AID, June 1978.

Anderson, M. A. and Grewal, Tina. "Nutrition Planning in the Developing World." Proceedings of regional workshops in India, Kenya, and Columbia. New York: CARE, 1977, p. 261.

Ashkenaz, Krishnamurthy, Thiagarajan, Moffat and Apta. Cultural Anthropology and Nutrition. Haverford, Pa.: Sidney M. Cantor Associates, 1973, P. 277.

Austin, J. E., ed. "Global Malnutrition and Cereal Fortification." Report submitted by Harvard University to AID, Washington, D. C., 1977, p. 179.

Baldwin, David A. Foreign Aid and American Foreign Policy. New York: Praeger, 1966.

Bauernfeind, J. G. "Vitamin A Technology and Xerophthalmia." Report to AID Office of Nutrition, Washington, D. C., 1973, 137 pp.

Burkhalter, B. R. "A Critical Review of Nutritional Planning Models and Experience." Community Systems Foundation report to AID Office of Nutrition, Washington, D. C., 1974.

Byrnes, Francis C. "Role Shock: An Occupational Hazard of American Technical Assistants Abroad," The Annals of the American Academy of Political and Social Science, vol. 368, November 1966.

Cole, Nick. "World Moves to Give Sight to Millions," Times of Indonesia, July 25, 1978.

Cook, T. M. "Planning National Nutrition Programs, A Suggested Approach." 2 vols. American Technical Assistance Corp. report to AID Office of Nutrition, Washington, D. C., 1973, vol. 1, 44 pp., vol. 2, 89 pp.

Crittenden, Ann. "The Realpolitik of Foreign Aid," The New York Times, February 26, 1978.

De Sagasti, H. E. E. and Hornik, R. C. "Communication and Education in Nutrition Planning in Costa Rica." Report to AID, Washington, D. C., 1975, 42 pp.

Fritz, Carl. "Battle against Blindness," War on Hunger (AID), vol. 11, no. 9, September-October, 1977.

Gershoff, McGandy, Gutta, Preyasri, "Nutrition Studies in Thailand. II. Effects of fortification of Rice with Lysine, Threomine, Thiamin, Riboflavin, Vitamin A and Iron on Preschool Children." The American Journal of Clinical Nutrition 30 (July 1977): 1185-95.

Helen Keller International. Periodic HKI Reports, New York.

Helen Keller International. The Right to See. New York: HKI, 1977.

Helen Keller International. Sixty Years of Caring about Blindness. New York: HKI, 1977.

Hirschman, Albert. Development Projects Observed. Washington, D. C.: The Brookings Institution, 1967.

Howard, Lee M. Key Problems Impeding Modernization of Developing Countries, the Health Issues. Washington, D. C.: AID, 1970, p. 55.

Hui, S. "Technical Application of Vitamin A." Paper presented to the Nutrition Research and Development Center in Bogor, Indonesia, February 1978, 7 pp.

Ingle, Marcus. Program Implementation in Developing Countries. Report to AID Office of Development Administration, Washington, D. C.: AID, March 1978, p. 56.

Ingle, Marcus. "Program Implementation Policies." Report to AID Office of Development Administration, Washington, D. C., April 1978, 32 pp.

Institute of Nutrition for Central America and Panama (INCAP). Fortification of Sugar with Vitamin A in Central America and Panama. Guatemala: INCAP, 1974, 39 pp.

Intech Inc. "Integrating Nutrition Planning Concerns into Agriculture and Health Sector Analysis." Report to AID, Washington, D. C., 1976, 138 pp.

International Agency for the Prevention of Blindness. Report of Xerophthalmia Group, First Assembly, July 5-9, 1978.

International Vitamin A Consultative Group. "Guidelines for the Eradication of Vitamin A Deficiency and Xerophthalmia." Report published by the Nutrition Foundation, New York: 1976.

Kamel, Wadie Wanies. "A Global Survey of Mass Vitamin A Programs." Report to AID Office of Nutrition, Washington, D. C., 1973, 56 pp.

Levinson, F. J. and Call, David L. "Nutrition Intervention in Low Income Countries: A Planning Model and Case Study." Cornell International Agricultural Development Mimeograph 34, 1970.

Majia, Hodges, Guillermo, Arroyave, Viteri and Tonin. "Vitamin A Deficiency and Anemia in Central American Children." The American Journal of Clinical Nutrition 30 (July 1977): 1175-84.

Manoff International Inc. "Using Modern Marketing Techniques for Nutrition Education." Report to AID Office of Nutrition, Washington, D. C., 1975, 173 pp.

Massachusetts Institute of Technology. Nutritional Program Development in Indonesia, MIT International Nutrition Planning Program. Technical Report Series no. 2. Cambridge: MIT, 1975.

Montgomery, John D. The Politics of Foreign AID. New York: Praeger, 1962, 336 pp.

Niblock, Thomas C. "What to Do about AID?" AID Forum, Washington, D. C., July 1978.

Raman, N. Pattabhi. "Project Implementation in the Context of a Plan: The Missing Links," Focus: Technical Cooperation, Washington, D. C.: Society for International Development, 1978 1.

Rasmuson, Mark. Current Practice and Future Directions of Nutrition Education in Developing Countries: A Research and Policy Assessment. Washington, D. C.: Academy for Educational Development for AID Offices of Nutrition and Education and Human Resources, 1977, 78 pp.

Rodinelli, Dennis A. "Implementing Development Projects: The Problem of Management," Focus: Technical Cooperation, Washington, D. C.: Society for International Development, 1978/1.

Rothman, Jack. Planning and Organizing for Social Change. New York: Columbia University Press, 1974.

Royston, Michael and Jordon, Victor. "Self Reliance and Environmental Management Education," Focus: Technical Cooperation, Washington, D. C.: Society for International Development, 1978/1.

Rubin, Emodi, and Scialpi. "Micronutrient Additions to Cereal Grain Products," Cereal Chemistry, vol. 54, no. 4, July-August 1977.

Smith, David and Mabel, Jessee. "Barriers between Expert and Counterpart," International Development Review (Society for International Development, Washington, D. C.), vol. 12, no. 1, 1970.

Solon, Fernandez, Latham and Popkin. "Research to Determine the Cause and Effectiveness of Alternate Means of Controlling Vitamin A Deficiency, and An Evaluation of Three Alternate Strategies to Prevent Xerophthalmia in the Philippines." Cornell University, 1977, 138 pp.

Solon, Popkin, Fernandez and Latham. "Vitamin A Deficiency in the Philippines: A Study of Xerophthalmia in Cebu." The American Journal of Clinical Nutrition 31 (February 1978): 360-68.

Sommer, A. Field Guide to the Detection and Control of Xerophthalmia. Geneva: World Health Organization, 1978, 49 pp.

Sommer, John G. Beyond Charity, U.S. Voluntary Aid for a Changing Third World. Washington, D.C.: Overseas Development Council, 1977, 180 pp.

Van Veen, Andre G., and Van Veen, Marjorie Scott. "Vitamin A Problems with Special Attention to Less Developed Countries." Report to AID Office of Nutrition, 1973, 62 pp.

Wolf, George. "A Historical Note on the Mode of Administration of Vitamin A for the Cure of Night Blindness." The American Journal of Clinical Nutrition 31 (February 1978): 290-2.

World Health Organization. "Vitamin A Deficiency and Xerophthalmia." Report of a Joint WHO/USAID Meeting, WHO Technical Report Series No. 590, Geneva, 1976, 98 pp.

Wilcke, H. L., ed. "Improving the Nutrient Quality of Cereals." Report of Second Workshop on Breeding and Fortification, September 12-17, 1976, convened by League for International Food Education for AID Offices of Nutrition and Agriculture, 332 pp.

Index

About the Author

CARL R. FRITZ is employed by the Government of Indonesia as an Advisor on nutrition management and planning. From 1977 to 1979, he was Liaison Officer for Helen Keller International, Nutritional Blindness Prevention Research Project in Indonesia. From 1973 to 1976, he was Director, Program Planning and Utilization, Technical Assistance Bureau, at AID in Washington, D.C. From 1970 to 1973, he was the Assistant Director of AID in Bangkok, and from 1969 to 1970 served as Deputy Associate Director of AID in Vietnam.

Pergamon Policy Studies

No. 1 Laszlo—*The Objectives of the New International Economic Order*
No. 2 Link/Feld—*The New Nationalism*
No. 3 Ways—*The Future of Business*
No. 4 Davis—*Managing and Organizing Multinational Corporations*
No. 5 Volgyes—*The Peasantry of Eastern Europe, Volume One*
No. 6 Volgyes—*The Peasantry of Eastern Europe, Volume Two*
No. 7 Hahn/Pfaltzgraff—*The Atlantic Community in Crisis*
No. 8 Renninger—*Multinational Cooperation for Development in West Africa*
No. 9 Stepanek—*Bangladesh—Equitable Growth?*
No. 10 Foreign Affairs—*America and the World 1978*
No. 11 Goodman/Love—*Management of Development Projects*
No. 12 Weinstein—*Bureaucratic Opposition*
No. 13 DeVolpi—*Proliferation, Plutonium and Policy*
No. 14 Francisco/Laird/Laird—*The Political Economy of Collectivized Agriculture*
No. 15 Godet—*The Crisis in Forecasting and the Emergence of the "Prospective" Approach*
No. 16 Golany—*Arid Zone Settlement Planning*
No. 17 Perry/Kraemer—*Technological Innovation in American Local Governments*
No. 18 Carman—*Obstacles to Mineral Development*
No. 19 Demir—*Arab Development Funds in the Middle East*
No. 20 Kahan/Ruble—*Industrial Labor in the U.S.S.R.*
No. 21 Meagher—*An International Redistribution of Wealth and Power*
No. 22 Thomas/Wionczek—*Integration of Science and Technology With Development*
No. 23 Mushkin/Dunlop—*Health: What Is It Worth?*
No. 24 Abouchar—*Economic Evaluation of Soviet Socialism*
No. 25 Amos—*Arab-Israeli Military/Political Relations*
No. 26 Geismar/Geismar—*Families in an Urban Mold*
No. 27 Leitenberg/Sheffer—*Great Power Intervention in the Middle East*
No. 28 O'Brien/Marcus—*Crime and Justice in America*
No. 29 Gartner—*Consumer Education in the Human Services*
No. 30 Diwan/Livingston—*Alternative Development Strategies and Appropriate Technology*
No. 31 Freedman—*World Politics and the Arab-Israeli Conflict*
No. 32 Williams/Deese—*Nuclear Nonproliferation*
No. 33 Close—*Europe Without Defense?*
No. 34 Brown—*Disaster Preparedness*

No. 35 Grieves—*Transnationalism in World Politics and Business*
No. 36 Franko/Seiber—*Developing Country Debt*
No. 37 Dismukes—*Soviet Naval Diplomacy*
No. 38 Morgan—*Science and Technology for Development*
No. 39 Chou/Harmon—*Critical Food Issues of the Eighties*
No. 40 Hall—*Ethnic Autonomy—Comparative Dynamics*
No. 41 Savitch—*Urban Policy and the Exterior City*
No. 42 Morris—*Measuring the Condition of the World's Poor*
No. 43 Katsenelinboigen—*Soviet Economic Thought and Political Power in the U.S.S.R*
No. 44 McCagg/Silver—*Soviet Asian Ethnic Frontiers*
No. 45 Carter/Hill—*The Criminal's Image of the City*
No. 46 Fallenbuchl/McMillan—*Partners in East-West Economic Relations*
No. 47 Liebling—*U.S. Corporate Profitability*
No. 48 Volgyes/Lonsdale—*Process of Rural Transformation*
No. 49 Ra'anan—*Ethnic Resurgence in Modern Democratic States*
No. 50 Hill/Utterback—*Technological Innovation for a Dynamic Economy*
No. 51 Laszlo/Kurtzman—*The United States, Canada and the New International Economic Order*
No. 52 Blazynski—*Flashpoint Poland*
No. 53 Constans—*Marine Sources of Energy*
No. 54 Lozoya/Estevez/Green—*Alternative Views of the New International Economic Order*
No. 55 Taylor/Yokell—*Yellowcake*
No. 56 Feld—*Multinational Enterprises and U.N. Politics*
No. 57 Fritz—*Combatting Nutritional Blindness in Children*
No. 58 Starr/Ritterbush—*Science, Technology and the Human Prospect*
No. 59 Douglass—*Soviet Military Strategy in Europe*
No. 60 Graham/Jordon—*The International Civil Service*
No. 61 Menon—*Bridges Across the South*
No. 62 Avery/Lonsdale/Volgyes—*Rural Change and Public Policy*
No. 63 Foster—*Comparative Public Policy and Citizen Participation*
No. 64 Laszlo/Kurtzman—*Eastern Europe and the New International Economic Order*
No. 65 United Nations Centre for Natural Resources, Energy and Transport—*State Petroleum Enterprises in Developing Countries*